§ 3.
med

11/36

RETROPERITONEOSCOPY

Edited by

Ara Darzi MD FRCS FRCSI
Consultant Surgeon, St Mary's Hospital, London
Senior Lecturer, St Mary's Hospital Medical School, Imperial College
 of Science and Technology
Tutor in Laparoscopic Surgery, Minimal Access Therapy Training Unit,
 Royal College of Surgeons in England
Honorary Consultant Surgeon, Central Middlesex Hospital, London

Illustrated by Dee McLean

I S I S
MEDICAL
MEDIA

Oxford

British Library Cataloguing in Publication Data
A catalogue record for this title is available from the British Library

ISBN 1 899066 29 2

Darzi A. (Ara)
Retroperitoneoscopy/
Ara Darzi

Always refer to the manufacturer's Prescribing Information
before prescribing drugs cited in this book

Typeset by
Creative Associates Ltd, Oxford, UK

Printed by
Printek S.A.L., Spain

Distributed by
Times Mirror International Publishers
Customer Service Centre, Unit 1, 3 Sheldon Way
Larkfield, Aylesford, Kent ME20 6SF, UK

Contents

List of Contributors

Giordano G. Abbondati MD
Consultant Anaesthetist, The Central Middlesex Hospital NHS Trust, Acton Lane, London NW10, UK

Martin J. Carney MD FACS
The Carney Center, 1868 Wildwood Drive, Virginia Beach, Virginia 23454, USA

Albert K. Chin MSME MD
Vice President of Research, Origin Medsystems Inc., 135 Constitution Drive, Menlo Park, California 94025, USA

Ara W. Darzi MD FRCS FRCSI
Consultant Surgeon, Academic Surgical Unit, S. Mary's Hospital Medical School, Praed Street, London W2 1NY, UK

Yves-Marie Dion MD MSc FRCSC FACS
Assistant Professor of Surgery, Laval University, Hôpital St. François d'Assise, 10 Rue De L'Espinay, Québec, G1L 3L5, Canada.

Jean-Louis Dulucq MD
Secretaire General, Société Française de Chirurgie Endoscopique, 203 route de Toulouse, MSP Bagatelle, 33401 Talence cedex, France

Durga D. Gaur MS FRCS(Eng)
Consultant Urological Surgeon and Associate Professor of Urology, Bombay Hospital, Institute of Medical Sciences, 19 Marine Lines, Bombay 400 020, India

Pierce A. Grace MCh FRCSI FRCS
Consultant Senior Lecturer in Vascular Surgery, Department of Surgery, Royal Postgraduate Medical School, Hammersmith Hospital, Du Cane Road, London W12 ONN, UK

Richard W. Graham MD
Urologist, Virginia Urology Center. Clinical Instructor of Surgery, Medical College of Virginia, Richmond, Virginia, USA

Jacques M. Himpens MD
University Hospital St. Pierre, 322 Hoogstraat, 1000 Brussels, Belgium

Pierre Hourlay MD
Abdominal Surgeon, Salvatorziekenhuis, Salvatorstraat 20, 3500 Hasselt, Belgium

Frederic H. Moll MD
Vice President and Medical Director, Origin Medsystems Inc., 135 Constitution Drive, Menlo Park, California, USA

Charles Nduka BA MBBS
Research Fellow, Minimal Access Surgery Unit, St. Mary's Hospital Medical School, Praed Street, London W2 1NY, UK

Paraskevas A. Paraskeva BSc(Hons) MBBS(Hons)
Surgical SHO, St. Mary's Hospital Medical School, Praed Street, London W2 1NY, UK

Michael Puttick BSc(Hons)
Honorary Research Fellow, Minimal Access Surgery Unit, St Mary's Hospital Medical School, Praed Street, London W2 1NY, UK

Helgi H. Sigurdsson CMCh FRCS FRCS(Ed)
Department of Surgery, Royal Postgraduate Medical School, Hammersmith Hospital, Du Cane Road, London W12 ONN, UK

Norman Silbertrust
Karl Storz Endovision, 91 Carpenter Hill Road, Charlton, MASS, 01507, USA

Richard J. Stacey MB BS FRCS
Registrar in Neurosurgery, Walton Centre for Neurology and Neurosurgery, Walton Hospital, Liverpool L9 1AE, UK

Geert G. Tailly MD
Urologist, Klina, Campus St. Jozef, Kerkstraat 9, B-2950 Kapellen, Belgium

Mark W. Wrigley MB BS FRCA
Consultant Anaesthetist, The Central Middlesex Hospital NHS Trust, Acton Lane, London NW10 7NS, UK

Preface

Minimal access surgical techniques have now expanded well beyond the initial innovation represented by laparoscopic cholecystectomy to encompass the broad range of procedures. Globally, millions of patients have benefitted. More importantly, however, it symbolises a change in the mind of General Surgeons from that of 'tradition followers' to that of 'innovative thinkers' willing to take the challenge of progress in a field of medicine which had grown staid.

The retroperitoneum has been described as a cemetery of medical reputations due to the difficulty in detecting and diagnosing disease in this area. Historically there has always been a debate over the relative merits of the retroperitoneal and the transperitoneal approaches to the retroperitoneal structures. Urologists have been the leaders in exploring this field and certainly John Wickham, one of the innovators of retroperitonoscopy described in 1987, the retroperitoneal insufflation with carbon dioxide and the use of a standard laparoscope to form the first endoscopic retroperitoneal ureterolithotomy. Because minimal access techniques in the retroperitoneum have truly been developed in a worldwide area, internationally renowned experts have been invited to contribute to this book. Moreover, because minimal access techniques to the retroperitoneum are used in various specialties, innovators in Vascular Surgery, Urology and General Surgery, have been asked to share their ideas and experiences.

Retroperitoneoscopy is part of perivisceral endoscopy, hence the inclusion of procedures which involve access in the absence of a natural cavity (i.e. endoscopic ligation of incompetent venous perforators and approaches to the breast and axilla).

An effort of this magnitude is of course not that of any individual but of many. I must express my appreciation for the highly professional and the enthusiastic manner which characterised our interaction with the staff of ISIS medical publishing. They have made the publication of this book a pleasure. I believe that the superb illustrations by Dee Maclean are one of the most outstanding aspects of this book. Finally, I would like to thank the authors of each chapter who have selflessly contributed their time and expertise to allow me to put together this comprehensive review of endoscopic retroperitoneal surgery.

Retroperitonoscopy presents a new frontier for minimal access surgery. I hope this book will provide a foundation for clinical judgement and assist others in further investigations to expand the application of minimally invasive surgery.

A Darzi

Chapter 1
Retroperitoneoscopy: history and background

M. Puttick, C.C. Nduka and A.W. Darzi

'There cannot always be fresh fields for conquest by the knife; there must be portions of the human frame that will ever remain sacred from intrusion at least in surgeons' hands.'
(John Eric Erichsen, 1873)

Early steps

The retroperitoneum has been described as the cemetery of medical reputations due to the difficulty in detecting and diagnosing disease in this area. Historically there has always been debate over the relative merits of the retroperitoneal and transperitoneal approaches to retroperitoneal structures. As early as 1878, Kocher performed an anterior transperitoneal nephrectomy through a midline incision. In 1913, Berg employed a transverse abdominal incision to mobilize the colon laterally to expose the great vessels and secure the renal pedicle. However, most urologists in the first half of this century adopted a retroperitoneal flank approach to the kidney, due to the high incidence of peritonitis and other abdominal complications. The development of safe abdominal and vascular surgical techniques during the late 1950s led to a revival of the anterior approach in patients undergoing renal surgery [1].

The first extraperitoneal approaches to the aorta were largely unsuccessful. In 1796, Abernathay failed attempting to ligate an external iliac artery aneurysm [2] and in 1874 a patient died 23 hours after Murray attempted a ligature of the abdominal aorta [3]. Two years later Sir Astley Cooper, using an extraperitoneal approach, successfully tied the external iliac artery in a man with a femoral aneurysm [4]. The first abdominal aortic aneurysm was resected in 1951 [5] and, in 1963, Rob described a series of 500 cases in which the aorta was approached by the retroperitoneal route [6]. Although transperitoneal repair of aortic aneurysms is the most widely applied technique today, several studies claim that the retroperitoneal approach to the aorta is clinically superior [7].

The advent of laparoscopic surgery has revolutionized surgery in the abdomen. As laparoscopic surgery has grown, so surgeons have been prompted to develop minimal access methods in other parts of the body. Minimal access approaches are, however, not a purely modern phenomenon. Bozzini is credited with the first recorded attempt at visualizing a body cavity when he created the 'Licht Leiter' in 1805 [8]. This was an awkward instrument used to visualize the urethra for stones and neoplasms. A light source was provided by a candle reflected by a series of mirrors. The provision of an adequate as well as practical light source remained a problem for the early endoscopists. Desormeaux used a device incorporating a kerosene lamp [9] and 2 years later Breslau examined a patient's mouth using an electrically heated platinum wire for illumination [10]. Obviously this device carried with it a significant risk of burn injuries. By the close of the 19th century many endoscopic devices were being used for a variety of open cavity procedures such as proctoscopy, laryngoscopy and oesophagoscopy. Devices now existed with parallel channels for surgical instruments. The first laparoscopies were reported by Ott [11], Kelling [12] and Jacobeus [13]. These early techniques involved inflating the abdomen with air to improve visualization but it was several years before the problem of creating a pneumoperitoneum was addressed.

Visualizing the space

A wide variety of instruments have been used in attempts to visualize the retroperitoneum. Rupel and Brown [14] used a cystoscope inserted though a nephrostomy track performed at open surgery to attempt a percutaneous renal stone removal. The first true retroperitoneoscopy was performed by Bartel in 1969 [15]. He used a short endoscope, similar to a mediastinoscope, inserted into the flank to inspect and examine the retroperitoneal space for the diagnosis of primary and secondary tumours in the retroperitoneum, retroperitoneal lymph node biopsy and lumbar sympathectomy.

Wittmoser employed a technique of blunt dissection with an endoscope and pneumatic dissection with carbon dioxide (CO_2) when performing an endoscopic lumbar sympathectomy in 1973 [16]. Fernstrom and Johnson described a radiological technique for percutaneous removal of renal stones in 1976 [17]. Wickham, in 1979, described retroperitoneal insufflation with carbon dioxide and the use of a standard laparoscope to perform the first endoscopic retroperitoneal ureterolithotomy [18].

Bay-Neilsen and Schultz removed stones from the upper half of the ureter in a series of six patients, visualizing the ureter with a laryngoscope [19]. A 3 cm long subcostal incision was made in the skin crease just lateral to the sacrospinal muscle. The peritoneum was pushed forward with a finger and the lower pole of the kidney felt and usually, the ureter with the stone in it as well. The laryngoscope was introduced and the ureter dissected. When mobilized, the ureter with stone was kinked up with a hook and the stone removed through a small incision. Stones were successfully removed in three out of six patients. Failures occurred because of inadequate instrumentation in the first case and large amounts of retroperitoneal fat in two obese patients.

In 1982 Fantoni *et al.* [20] used a mediastinoscope inserted under local anaesthetic to perform 'low' retroperitoneoscopy. This technique was so-called because with a short mediastinoscope inserted between the anterior superior iliac spine and the pubic tubercle, the exploration was limited to unilateral exploration at a level below the aortic bifurcation. Blunt dissection under direct vision using the tip of the instrument was employed, freeing the fascia over the iliopsoas and exposing the external iliac artery and associated lymph nodes. On-table screening lymphography was used to direct the instrument towards the desired lymph nodes. Pathological tissue and lymph nodes were biopsied and bleeding controlled by diathermy. These were isolated attempts and it is only now that we realize their significance. The advantages of minimal access surgery (shorter hospital stay, early return to work, less postoperative pain, fewer wound complications and cosmetically better scars) have recently become apparent and are well documented [21–28]. It now seems only logical that laparoscopic experience should be applied in other fields of surgery.

Current perspectives

Modern advances in endoscopic technology have meant that the new cameras can produce ever-improving picture quality. Conventional laparoscopic equipment can be used to visualize the retroperitoneal space. One factor that has until recently prevented the growth in retroperitoneoscopic surgery from paralleling that of laparoscopic surgery has been the ability to create space. Unlike the abdomen, the retroperitoneum is a potential space rather than an actual space so there must be space created in which the surgeon can work. The first technique used was insufflation of carbon dioxide. Retroperitoneal insufflation of gas was first developed as a pneumographic technique for outlining the kidney and adrenal glands to allow radiographic definition of renal and adrenal tumours [29,30]. This procedure is no longer used as a radiographic technique because more sensitive and less invasive tests are now available. Difficulty in achieving a satisfactory pneumoretroperitoneum that could break down the dense areolar tissue binding the fat in the retroperitoneum led to the dissection being performed endoscopically [31].

Gaur, working in Bombay, did a lot to overcome these problems. He pioneered the design of a balloon dissector which consisted of a size 7 surgeon's glove tied on to the end of a urinary catheter and inflated with the bulb of a sphygmomanometer [32]. Following a skin incision just above the iliac crest and blunt dissection, the balloon was inserted into the retroperitoneal space. The balloon was inflated until a bulge appeared in the abdomen with a maximum pressure of about 110 mmHg. This decreased to 40–50 mmHg as the septae were broken down. The balloon was left in place for 5 minutes to achieve haemostasis, deflated and removed. Carbon dioxide was then insufflated through a laparoscopic port and the procedure performed. Gaur has recently modified this technique to allow simultaneous laparoscopic dissection as well as retroperitoneal dissection. This is achieved by inserting the laparoscope inside a condom balloon [33].

McDougall modified Gaur's technique by filling the finger of a surgeon's glove with saline [34]. The use of saline should reduce the risk of trauma to the retroperitoneum should the balloon burst. We have devised a 'balloon laparoscope' by placing a modified endotracheal tube over a laparoscope and we have successfully used it in endoscopic varicose veins surgery, colonic mobilization and hiatus hernia surgery. There are now specially designed balloon trocars into which a laparoscope can be inserted [35]. With the balloon in place the dissection can be observed.

Retroperitoneoscopy has since been used to perform surgery on many retroperitoneal structures. Percutaneous removal of the kidney began in 1988 when Smith and co-workers attempted to remove a pig kidney by means of a single tract, percutaneous approach [36]. Their sole laboratory experience was complicated by a colonic injury and the project was abandoned. Ikari et al. [37] also reported a single clinical case in which an attempt was made to remove a non-functioning kidney by a single tract, percutaneous approach. The renal artery was embolized and the renal parenchymal tissue was avulsed by grasping forceps and delivered through the nephrostomy tract. A total of 16 g of tissue was removed but postoperative sonography showed that about 17 g of tissue remained in place. Clayman *et al.* [38,39] were prompted to examine the feasibility of a minimal access approach to nephrectomy following the development of laparoscopic technology and techniques. Initially, almost all laparoscopic nephrectomies were performed with a transperitoneal approach. Following placement of five entry ports, the kidney was dissected, the renal vessels and ureter clipped and the kidney manoeuvred into a specially designed organ entrapment sack. The neck of the sack was brought to the surface of the abdomen at the umbilical port site and the kidney morcellated and the fragments aspirated with a high speed electrical tissue morcellator. The empty sack was then pulled from the abdomen.

Laparoscopic nephrectomy for benign disease has become increasingly accepted by surgeons [40,41] but laparoscopic nephroureterectomy and nephrectomy for malignant disease remain controversial for two main reasons. Firstly, and most importantly, there is a potential for tumour seeding at the time of tissue morcellation and organ retrieval. Secondly, tissue morcellation prevents histological analysis of the kidney to accurately grade and stage the tumour. Both these problems can be overcome by the current practice of entrapping the diseased kidney and removing it intact via a 5–7 cm incision. Living donor nephrectomy performed retroperitoneoscopically has recently been reported in two patients [42].

The retroperitoneal location of the adrenal glands renders them relatively inaccessible for a transabdominal laparoscopic approach, particularly because of their high cephalad position and the overlying colon, liver, spleen and pancreas. The first retroperitoneoscopic attempts at adrenalectomy were peformed in the pig using insufflation of the retroperitoneal space with carbon dioxide and retroperitoneoscopy [43]. One pig died from a right-side pneumothorax attributable to penetration with a trocar but six pigs recovered uneventfully from the procedure. Autopsies peformed 37–51 days postoperatively showed minimal scarring of the adrenalectomy bed. Uchida *et al.* [44] performed retroperitoneoscopic adrenalectomy in six patients in cases of primary aldosteronism. The treatment was successful in all cases with one occurrence of pneumothorax.

Laparoscopic colonic surgery has not developed at the same rate as other procedures. This is largely due to concerns about potential risks of laparoscopic surgery for neoplasia as well as the requirement for advanced laparoscopic skills and deficiencies in instrumentation. Stacey *et al.* [45] describe a retroperitoneal approach to both laparoscopic and open colonic mobilization (right, left and rectal) using a specially designed distension balloon. Transparent balloons allow constant visualization during distension via a video laparoscope inserted into the balloon port. The colon and its mesentery were mobilized from their retroperitoneal attachments and they obtained close views of the ureters, gonadal vessels and duodenum in right-sided mobilization. This approach also has the potential advantage, in cases of colectomy for neoplasia, of mobilizing the mesenteric vessels down to their origin. To perform the procedure with extra safety, simultaneous laparoscopy with an additional endoscope is employed. If the initial laparoscopy found a tumour to be fixed then an open approach could easily be adopted.

Wurtz in 1989 reported the results of 135 retroperitoneoscopies in 106 patients performed over 3 years [46]. In this series the diagnostic accuracy of retroperitoneoscopy (94%) was superior to that of other diagnostic investigations and in many cases eliminated the need for exploratory laparotomy. Villers *et al.* [47], in France, performed endoscopic lymph node dissection with CO_2 insufflation of the retroperitoneal space in 30 patients as part of the staging of prostate and bladder cancers. With conventional laparoscopic equipment they performed complete bilateral dissection of the ilio-obturator lymph nodes in 24 cases (80%). In six cases only unilateral dissection was performed because of technical complications such as venous injury. In the patients who subsequently underwent radical operations no intraoperative or postoperative morbidity relating to endoscopic lymph node dissection was observed.

There are other literature reports of retroperitoneoscopy being used for diagnosis of lymphogenic metastases of bladder cancer [48], metastatic and primary retroperitoneal tumours [49], skin melanoma metastases in the iliac lymph nodes [50] and anatomical assessment of retroperitoneal adenopathies [51]. Zhila *et al.* [52] used a retroperitoneoscope for high ligation and transection of the testicular vein in 90 young males suffering from left-sided varicocele with no intraoperative complications and no recurrence with a follow-up of 2 years.

Potential pitfalls

Retroperitoneoscopy offers several advantages over the transabdominal laparoscopic approach [43]. The retroperitoneal approach is more direct, obviating the need for laparoscopic dissection of the overlying colon, liver, spleen and pancreas which can be both tedious and time consuming. Conversely there are disadvantages. The view of the anatomy can be disorientating for the inexperienced surgeon or for the laparoscopic surgeon accustomed to viewing the abdomen and retroperitoneum from an anterior, transabdominal position. The working space in the retroperitoneum is small and limits the number of working ports that can be inserted as well as the dissection angles. Observing the movements of long instruments on a two-dimensional screen leads to problems with hand–eye coordination, depth perception and tactile sensory feedback. As with other branches of minimally invasive surgery, training courses should be attended.

Insufflation of the retroperitoneum has the potential for complications including CO_2 embolism and mediastinal emphysema (pneumothorax and pneumomediastinum) [43]. There are only isolated reports of mediastinal emphysema that have resulted from inadvertent insufflation of the retroperitoneum of non-CO_2 gases during colonoscopy [53], culdoscopy [54] and fulguration of bladder tumours [55]. The presumed mechanism of mediastinal emphysema development is thought to involve dissection of air or gas from the retroperitoneum into the chest via small openings in the diaphragm or via the aortic or oesophageal hiatus [56,57], but whether these potential openings become clinically significant when rapidly absorbed CO_2 gas is used to insufflate the retroperitoneum is unknown. The low frequency of this in the pre-computed tomography scan era of presacral and retroperitoneal pneumography is evidence against this and risks of pneumomediastinum and pneumothorax in humans should be low, especially when patients are receiving positive pressure ventilation [42]. Pneumomediastinum has also been reported following laparoscopic Nissen fundoplication.

The future

The history of retroperitoneoscopic surgery is one of innovation, lateral thinking and technological advance. Innovation, where new instruments have been designed and new surgical techniques developed, lateral thinking in the application of existing technology to new problems and in novel ways, and technological advance in the fields of instrument design and video endoscopy have allowed the rapid development of a totally new and exciting branch of surgery. The evolution of all minimally invasive therapies has been inextricably linked to technological advances which serve to miniaturize our eyes, extend our hands and allow surgery to be performed in places previously reached only by large incisions. Retroperitoneoscopy has been used in many areas of surgical practice. These include ureterolithotomy, nephrectomy, adrenalectomy, lumbar sympathectomy, staging and biopsy of cancers and lymph nodes, colonic mobilization and ligation of the testicular vein in varicoceles. In the future we believe that there will be other uses including the removal of undescended testicles, pancreatic biopsy, aortic surgery and lumbar discectomy. Retroperitoneoscopy is a minimal access technique which has developed as a result of the technical and technological progress made in laparoscopic surgery. Techniques are undergoing continual modification [58] and we are only now beginning to realize the potentials of retroperitoneoscopy. In some cases retroperitoneoscopy is a viable alternative to laparoscopy or open surgery. It is important, however, that before this technique is accepted, controlled trials are undertaken and more technical developments are made. Nevertheless, as minimal access techniques continue to evolve, we will undoubtedly see more parts of the body enter the reach of the surgeon.

'Law number six: there is no body cavity that cannot be reached with a number fourteen needle and a good strong arm'.
(Samuel Shem. In: *The House of God*. London: Black Swan, 1978: p85.)

References

1   Novich AC, Streem SB. Surgery of the kidney. In: Walsh PC, Ketick AB, Stamey TA, Darracott Vaughn E Jr (eds) *Campbell's Urology*, Vol. 3, 6th edn. Philadelphia: WB Saunders, 1993: 2413–500.
2   Abernathay J. In: *Surgical Observations*. London: Longman and O'Rees, 1804; 209–31.
3   Anon. Dr Murray's case of ligature of the abdominal aorta. *Ann R Coll Surg Engl* 1984; **66**: 408.
4   Cooper A. Case of femoral artery aneurysm for which the external iliac artery was tied by Sir Astley Cooper. Taken from Sir Astley Cooper's notes. *Guy's Hosp Rep* 1836; **1**: 43–52.
5   Dubost C, Allary M, Oeconomos N. Resection of an aneurysm of the abdominal aorta. *Arch Surg* 1952; **64**: 405–8.
6   Rob C. Extraperitoneal approach to the abdominal aorta. *Surg* 1963; **53**: 87–9.
7   Grace PA, Bouchier-Hayes D. Infrarenal abdominal aortic disease: a review of the retroperitoneal approach. *Br J Surg* 1991; **78**: 6–9.
8   Bozzini P. Lichtleiter, eine Erfindung Zur Anschung Innerer Theile und Krankheiten Nebst Abbildung. *J Pract Arzehunde* 1806; **24**: 107.
9   Desormeaux AJ. Transactions of the Société de Chirurgie, Paris. Gazette des Hopitale 1865, 16.
10 Belt AE, Charnock DA. The history of the cystoscope. In: Cabot H (ed) *Modern Urology*. Philadelphia: Lea & Febiger, 1936: 15.
11 Ott D. Illumination of the abdomen (ventroscopia) [Russian]. *J. Akush I Zhensk* 1901; **15**: 1045.
12 Kelling G. Uber Oesophagoskopie. Gastroskopie und Koelioskopie. *Munich Med Wochenschr* 1901; **49**: 21.
13 Jacobeus HC. Uber die Moglichkeit: die Zystoskopie bei Untersuchung serser Hohlungen anzuwenden. *Munich Med Wochenschr* 1910; **57**: 2090–2.

14 Rupel DE, Brown R. Nephroscopy with removal of stone following nephrostomy for obstructive calculus anuria. *J Urol* 1941; **46**: 177.

15 Bartel M. Die Retroperitoneoskopie. Eine endoskopische Methode zur Inspektion und bioptischen Untersuchung des retroperitonealen Raumes. *Zentralbl Chir* 1969; **94**: 377–83.

16 Wittmoser R. Die Retroperitoneoskopie als neue Methode der lumbalen Sympathikotomie. *Fortschr Endosk* 1973; **4**: 219–23.

17 Fernstrom I, Johnson B. Percutaneous puncture nephrostomy. In: Anderson *et al.* (eds) *Encyclopedia of Urology*, Vol 1. Berlin: Springer-Verlag, 1976.

18 Wickham JEA. The surgical treatment of renal lithiasis. In: Wickham JEA (ed) *Urinary Calculous Disease*, New York: Churchill-Livingstone, 1979; 145–98.

19 Bay-Neilsen H, Schultz A. Endoscopic retroperitoneal removal of stones from the upper half of the ureter. *Scand J Urol Nephrol* 1982; **16**: 227–8.

20 Fantoni PA, Tognoli S, Astuni M *et al.* A technique of low retroperitoneoscopy. *Endoscopy* 1982; **14**: 102–4.

21 Dubios F, Icard P, Berthelot G, Levard H. Celioscopic cholecystectomy. *Ann Surg* 1990; **211**: 60–3.

22 Grace PA, Quereshi A, Coleman J *et al.* Reduced post operative hospitalisation after laparoscopic cholecystectomy. *Br J Surg* 1991; **78**: 160–2.

23 Graves HA Jr, Ballinger JF, Anderson WJ. Appraisal of laparoscopic cholecystectomy. *Ann Surg* 1991; **213**: 655–64.

24 Peters JH, Ellison EC, Innes JT *et al.* Safety and efficacy of laparoscopic cholecystectomy. *Ann Surg* 1991; **213**: 3–12.

25 Schirmer BD, Edge SB, Dix J *et al.* Laparoscopic cholecystectomy. *Ann Surg* 1992; **216**: 146–52.

26 Spaw AT, Reddick E, Olsen D. Laparoscopic laser cholecystectomy: analysis of 500 procedures. *Surg Laparosc Endosc* 1991; **1**: 2–7.

27 Southern Surgeons Club. A prospective analysis of 1518 laparoscopic cholecystectomies. *N Engl J Med* 1991; **324**: 1073–8.

28 Wastell C. Laparoscopic cholecystectomy: better for patients and the health service (editorial). *Br Med J* 1991; **302**: 304–5.

29 Sowerbutts JG. Some uses for presacral oxygen insufflation. *J Fac Radiol* 1959; **10**: 201–6.

30 Saxton HM, Strickland B. Presacral pneumography. In: (eds) *Practical Procedures in Diagnostic Radiology*, 2nd edn. London: HK Lewis, 1972: 160–8.

31 Wickham JEA, Miller RA. Percutaneous renal access. In: Miller RA (ed) *Percutaneous Renal Surgery*. New York: Churchill Livingstone, 1983; 33–9.

32 Gaur DD. Laparoscopic operative retroperitoneoscopy: use of a new device. *J Urol* 1992; **148**: 1137–9.

33 Gaur DD *et al.* Laparoscopic condom dissection: new technique of retroperitoneoscopy. *J Endourol* 1994; **8**: 149–51.

34 McDougall EM, Clayman RV, Fadden PT. Retroperitoneoscopy: the Washington University Medical School experience. *Urology* 1994; **43**: 446–52.

35 Hirsch IH, Moreno JG, Lotfi MA, Gomella LG. Controlled balloon dilation of the extraperitoneal space for laparoscopic urologic surgery. *J Laparoendosc Surg* 1994; **4**: 247–51.

36 Weinberg JJ, Smith AD. Percutaneous resection of the kidney: preliminary report. *J Endourol* 1988; **2**: 355–61.

37 Ikari O, Netto NT Jr, Palma PCR, D'Ancona CA. Percutaneous nephrectomy in nonfunctioning kidneys: a preliminary report. *J Urol* 1990; **144**: 966–8.

38 Clayman RV, Kavoussi LR, Long SL *et al.* Laparoscopic nephrectomy: initial report of pelviscopic organ ablation in the pig. *J Endourol* 1990; **4**: 247–52.

39 Clayman RV, Kavoussi LR, Soper NJ *et al.* Laparoscopic nephrectomy: review of the initial 10 cases. *J Endourol* 1992; **6**: 127–32.

40 Kerbl K, Figenshau RS, Clayman RV *et al.* Retroperitoneal laparoscopic nephrectomy: laboratory and clinical experience. *J Endourol* 1993a; **7**: 23–6.

41 Kerbl K, Clayman RV, McDougall EM, Kavoussi LR. Laparoscopic nephrectomy. *Br Med J* 1993b; **307**: 1488–9.

42 Yang SC, Lee DH, Rha KH, Park K. Retroperitoneoscopic living donor nephrectomy: two cases. *Transplant Proc* 1994; **26**: 2409.

43 Brunt LM, Molmenti EP, Kerbl K, Soper NJ, Stone MS, Clayman RV. Retroperitoneal endoscopic adrenalectomy: an experimental study. *Surg Laparosc Endosc* 1993; **3**: 300–6.

44 Uchida M, Imaide Y, Yoneda K *et al.* Endoscopic adrenalectomy by retroperitoneal approach for primary aldosteronism. *Hinyokika Kiyo* 1994; **40**: 43–6.

45 Stacey R, Hunt N, Darzi A. Retroperitoneoscopy and retroperitoneal colonic mobilisation: a new approach in laparoscopic colonic surgery. *Br J Surg* 1995; **82**: 1038–9.

46 Wurtz A. L'endoscopie de l'espace retroperitoneal. Techniques, resultats et indications actuelles. *Ann Chir* 1989; **43**: 475–80.

47 Villers A, Abecassis R, Baron JC *et al.* Curage ganglionnaire endoscopique extra-peritoneal avec insufflation dans le bilan d'extension des cancers vesicaux et protatiques. *Prog Urol* 1992; **2**: 892–900.

48 Matveev BP, Shipilov VI, Ali-Zade AM. Retroperitoneoskopiia v diagnostikeä limfogennylh metastozov mochevogo puzyria. *Vopr Onkol* 1984; **30**: 87–90.

49 Knysh VI, Cherkes VL, Tsariuk VF. Retroperitoneoskopiia v diagnostikeä metastaticheskikh i pervichnykh zabriushinnykh opukholei. *Khirurgiia (Mosk)* 1982; **5**: 71–3.

50 Vagner RI, Tarkov AS, Kolosov AE, Matytsin AN. Retroperitoneopelvioskopiia v diagnostike metastazov melanomy kozhi v povzdoshnye limfaticheskie uzly. *Vestn Khir* 1986; **137**: 99–100.

51 Wurtz A, Mazeman E, Gosselin B, Woelffle D, Sauvage L, Rousseau O. Bilan anatomique des adenopathies retroperitoneales par endoscopie chirurgicale. A propos de 52 retroperitoneoscopies chez 49 malades. *Ann Chir* 1987; **41**: 258–63.

52 Zhila VV, Shodmonova ZR, Rublevskii VP, Chernenko PS. Vysokaia rezektsiia levoi veny iaichka i pereviazka vnutrennikh podvzdoshnykh arterii s pomoshchiuä retroperitoneoskopa. *Klin Khir* 1991; **5**: 49–51.

53 Schmidt G, Borsch G, Wegener M. Subcutaneous emphysema and pneumothorax complicating diagnostic colonoscopy. *Dis Colon Rectum* 1986; **29**: 136–8.

54 Fortier QE. Retroperitoneal, mediastinal and cervical emphysema following culdoscopy. *Fertil Steril* 1954; **5**: 173–81.

55 Sivak BJ. Surgical emphysema: report of a case and review. *Anesth Analg* 1964; **43**: 415–17.

56 Rivas MR. Roentgenological diagnosis: generalised subserous emphysema through a single puncture. *Am J Roentgenol* 1950; **64**: 723–34.

57 Joannides M, Tsoulos GD. The etiology of interstitial and mediastinal emphysema. *Arch Surg* 1930; **21**: 333–9.

58 Rassweiler JJ, Henkel TO, Stock CH *et al*. Retroperitoneal laparoscopic nephrectomy and other procedures in the upper retroperitoneum using a balloon dissection technique. *Eur Urol* 1994; **25**: 229–36.

Chapter 2
Anaesthesia for major abdominal laparoscopic surgery

M.W. Wrigley and G.G. Abbondati

'Do no harm' (Hippocrates 460–370 BC)

Introduction

The duty of the anaesthetist to the patient is to prevent the patient from coming to harm during surgery. At the present time laparoscopic surgery is performed better by some than others. The anaesthetist must sometimes be prepared to insist that the open procedure is substituted in the interest of the patient. The relationship between the surgeon and anaesthetist is of paramount importance. There must be a mutual understanding of what is proposed to be performed and both parties must anticipate the potential problems that each may encounter. Good and honest communication is the key to safe anaesthesia and surgery. The anaesthetist who allows an unwell patient to be operated on by an untrained surgeon doing an unwise procedure is a responsible as the surgeon when things go wrong.

Physiology

The introduction of gas into the abdominal cavity has significant effects on many aspects of normal physiology.

Respiratory physiology

The upward displacement and splinting of the diaphragm leads to an increase in the work of breathing and the potential of basal collapse of the lungs. The peak airway pressure and plateau pressure rise by 50% and 81%, whilst the compliance falls by 47% [1].

The use of carbon dioxide (CO_2) gas causes absorption of CO_2 to the tune of 70 ml/min for the first 30 minutes and 90 ml/min after this [2]. Hence there is an increase in the need to excrete CO_2. The only safe way of resolving this is to overventilate the lungs using controlled positive pressure ventilation, with a raised minute volume, in such a way as to clear the extra CO_2 [3,4] and to hold open the basal segments of the lungs.

Occasionally patients will have respiratory disease where they will retain CO_2 during surgery. Oxygenation is not normally a problem [5]. Preoperative pulmonary function tests showing decreased flow of, for example, forced expiratory volume (FEV_1), forced vital capacity (FVC), etc. and impaired diffusion are predictors for intraoperative acidosis [6]. Normally with controlled ventilation this is manageable, although with extraperitoneal dissection, where more gas is absorbed [7,8], the minute ventilation rates may have to be further increased to a level that imposes constraints on airway pressure and expiratory time. In these cases, possible solutions include attempts to perform the surgery at a lower insufflation pressure, the use of a gasless method using a mechanical retractor [9–11] or the use of an alternative gas such as helium [12,13] or argon [14,15]. Ultimately an open procedure may have to be substituted.

A rare complication of pneumoperitoneum is that of pneumothorax and the anaesthetist must be prepared to recognize and treat this [16].

Laparoscopic cholecystectomy causes a residual depression in respiratory parameters, compliance remaining depressed after pneumoperitoneum [1] and FEV_1 and FVC still being 22% and 23% depressed 24 hours after surgery [17]. This depression is, however, less than would be expected following open surgery [18].

It is mandatory to measure end-tidal CO_2 levels during surgery as these correlate well with arterial levels [2,19].

Cardiovascular physiology

The most profound effect of pneumoperitoneum seen by the anaesthetist is an increase in the blood pressure and, therefore, the mean arterial pressure (MAP) [20], often accompanied by a tachycardia [21]. However, vagal effects of distension can occasionally cause significant bradycardia. Cardiac output studies using thermodilution techniques and oesophageal Doppler methods show complex and alarming changes in haemodynamics which are independent of the gas used [15].

The pneumoperitoneum compresses the blood vessels in the abdomen leading to pooling of blood in the legs and a decrease in the amount of blood in the abdominal venous system. Both the central venous pressure (CVP) and pulmonary capillary wedge pressure (PAOP) increase but this is not associated with an increase in cardiac output as would be expected [22] and normally a 25% fall in cardiac index occurs [15]. Because of this an increase in the oxygen extraction ratio is to be expected and hence the mixed venous oxygen saturation falls [5]. This fall in cardiac index is because the external pressure of the pneumoperitoneum on the abdominal arterial circulation causes an increase in afterload [23] that raises the resistance that the left ventricle has to overcome. The magnitude of the intra-abdominal pressure induced by the pneumoperitoneum affects this [24].

The degree of patient tilt affects the cardiac filling pressures. A horizontal position and pneumoperitoneum leads to increases of 58% in CVP, 32% in PAOP and 39% in MAP. A 20° head-down tilt is associated with a further 40% increase in filling pressures. A 20° head-up tilt will reduce the filling pressures to the pre-pneumoperitoneum levels. The increased afterload is maintained in both head-up and head-down tilts [22].

These adverse haemodynamic effects do not preclude surgery on poor-risk patients, but aggressive haemodynamic monitoring is needed for such patients [20]. Pneumoperitoneum has been found to cause pulmonary oedema in a patient with impaired left ventricular function (M. Wrigley & G.G. Abbondati, unpublished data). In a hypovolaemic trauma patient, a pneumoperitoneum may cause haemodynamic changes beyond the compensatory capacity of the cardiovascular system [23]. Adequate crystalloid resuscitation does not decrease the risk of this [25]. Occasionally, cardiovascular collapse has occurred [26]. The first response to this should be immediate deflation of the pneumoperitoneum.

To summarize, the cardiovascular physiology comprises the following:

1 Venous pooling in the legs.
2 Decreased arterial and venous blood volume in the abdomen.
3 An increase in CVP and PAOP.
4 Increased left ventricular afterload.
5 Decreased cardiac output.

Central nervous system physiology

Laparoscopic surgery is unwise in the presence of intracranial injuries because the pneumoperitoneum will decrease the cerebral perfusion pressure (CPP). The CPP is the difference between the MAP (which rises) and the CVP (which also rises) minus the intracranial pressure (ICP). The ICP rises with the pneumoperitoneum due to a raised CVP and this can affect the CPP [27]. Head-down tilt and intracranial space-occupying lesions will exacerbate these effects. In these cases it is preferable to use open operation or gasless techniques. We predict that there will be a case of report of a patient underoging laparoscopic bowel surgery in a steep head-down tilt, with an undiagnosed cerebral metastasis, suffering a significant intracranial event.

The effect of increased venous pressure on the eyes is yet to prove a problem but it potentially worrying as venous return from the retina is embarrassed.

Renal physiology

The effect of pneumoperitoneum on renal function is a decrease in the creatinine clearance rate [28]. This is as a result of the generalized decrease in splanchnic flow found during pneumoperitoneum [24]. This is translated into a decreased urine flow during surgery, especially in patients with pre-existing cardiac disease [29].

Complications

Venous pooling

Pneumoperitoneum causes pooling in the venous system of the legs. There is both a distension of the veins and a decrease in the flow velocity in the large veins of the lower limbs [30]. Low dose heparin in conjunction with external compression devices will reduce the risk of deep vein thrombosis [31], although at insufflation pressures above 12 mmHg decreases in venous flow cannot be completely reversed [30]. Early ambulation may, however, lead to a lower venous thrombosis rate [17].

Metabolic

All operations cause a stress response but these are more reduced after laparoscopic surgery than after open surgery [17]. Prolonged insufflation may cause a rise in potassium levels.

Temperature

During laparoscopic surgery CO_2 is insufflated into the peritoneal cavity. This gas is stored as a liquid and in the process of evaporation becomes cold. As a result the patient is cooled to the extent of 0.3° per 50 litres of gas insufflated [33]. Warming the gas can obviate this [34].

Sickle cell anaemia

The anaesthetic goals in sickle cell anaemia are a warm, well-hydrated and well-perfused patient with full oxygenation. The fall in temperature [33], low cardiac output [15], high oxygen extraction ration [5] and venous pooling [30] will mitigate against this. The authors feel that prolonged pneumoperitoneum is inadvisable in this condition.

Operative complications

The introduction of the initial insufflation needle can cause perforation of any of the intra-abdominal organs. A gastric tube is mandatory for any upper abdominal work and probably for all abdominal laparoscopic surgery. This must be placed under suction before surgery starts. Our preference is to insert an orogastric tube in all patients for which a long-term tube is unnecessary.

End-tidal CO_2 sampling will rapidly demonstrate a CO_2 embolus [35]; a sudden drop in end-tidal CO_2 excretion is indicative of massively reduced pulmonary perfusion caused by gas bubbles in the circulation. The treatment of this is to stop insufflating and to use standard methods for the treatment of an air embolism.

Prophylactic antibiotics should cover minor inadvertent bowel perforation, but laparoscopic surgery is unwise in the presence of obstructive bowel disease.

Nitrous oxide will diffuse into any gas-filled spaces and its use is questionable in prolonged abdominal cases.

Anaesthetic technique

The authors feel that to prescribe a recipe for anaesthesia for laparoscopic surgery is unwise and potentially arrogant. We see the patient preoperatively, paying particular attention to the respiratory and cardiac reserve. If there are any pre-existing respiratory conditions we insist on investigations of pulmonary function, and for all patients with a cardiac history we would like, at the least, an electrocardiogram (ECG) and possibly a cardiological opinion as well. Premedication in our unit is minimal — a short-acting benzodiazepine such as temazepam being the most that we use.

Anaesthetic induction consists of a combination of a short-acting opiate (fentanyl), droperidol for its α-adrenergic blocking effects and antiemetic actions, an intravenous induction agent (propofol for quick cases and thiopentone for longer cases) and a non-depolarizing muscle relaxant (vecuronium). We ventilate the patient with an oral endotraceal tube and pass a nasogastric or orogastric tube and aspirate it. In lower abdominal operations a catheter must be placed in the bladder before surgery commences. We site a large bore (14 gauge) intravenous cannula. In major bowel resections we site a CVP line mainly to assist the postoperative fluid management. We use epidurals only on combined laparoscopic and open operations. The patient is ventilated with oxygen, nitrous oxide and isoflurane; the isoflurane decreases the left ventricular afterload. Nitrous oxide is omitted in major bowel resections and in potentially long cases where we use oxygen, air and isoflurane instead. Perioperative analgesia is provided either with increments of fentanyl or morphine. Particular emphasis is placed on the safe positioning of the patient.

Prophylactic cephalosporins are administered to all patients who are not allergic to them; in the presence of allergy an alternative is used. Where mesh is to be inserted, antibiotic cover is very important. In major bowel surgery metronidazole is added. Deep venous thrombosis prophylaxis is very important in all cases. Monitoring of the patient consists of an ECG and measurements of end-tidal CO_2, non-invasive blood pressure, airway pressure, pulse oximetry, inspired and expired oxygen and vapour and a disconnection alarm.

Good muscle relaxation allows the surgeon to have good vision of the intra-abdominal organs with a low insufflation pressure. Minimally invasive surgery occurs in a darkened room with a covered patient so the role of the anaesthetist is to look after *the patient* and not to admire the surgery being performed on the television screen.

We administer intramuscular opiates during the procedure so that the patient has an adequate level of postoperative analgesia. The surgeon should remove as much gas as possible from the peritoneal space as this significantly decreases postoperative pain [36]. Instillation of fluid [37] or local anaesthetic (M. Wrigley & G.G. Abbondati, unpublished data) can also decrease postoperative pain. Non-steroidal anti-inflammatory agents are of use postoperatively, but we are cautious of their use with asthmatic patients and avoid them altogether in patients with pre-existing renal disease. Their action on platelet function remains a concern.

At the end of the surgery we reverse the muscle relaxation and transfer the patient to the recovery ward. We prescribe intermittent intramuscular opiates as we find that few patients need patient-controlled analgesia. Antiemetics are prescribed. Patients with severe pain are treated with intravenous opioids until the pain is gone. Small doses of benzodiazepines can help with this. We find that this period of acute postoperative pain following pneumoperitoneum is rare and the acute need for opiates reduces rapidly following the termination of surgery. The patients usually are in hospital over the night following surgery but patients with good social backup may be discharged earlier. Severe continuing pain which is unresponsive to opiates is a cause for concern as in our experience it may be related to continuing bleeding or peritonitis.

References

1   Bardoczky GI, Engleman E, Levarlet M, Simon P. Ventilatory effects of pneumoperitoneum monitored with continuous spirometry. *Anaesthesia* 1993; **48**(4): 309–11.
2   Wurst H, Schulte-Steinberg H, Finsterer U. Pulmonary CO_2 elimination in laparoscopic cholecystectomy. A clinical study (in German). *Anaesthesist* 1993; **42**(7): 427–34.

3   Tan PL, Lee TL, Tweed WA. Carbon dioxide absorption and gas exchange during pelvic laparoscopy. *Can J Anaesth* 1992; **39**(7): 677–81.

4   Walsh MT, Vetter TR. Anesthesia for pediatric laparoscopic cholecystectomy. *J Clin Anesth* 1992; **4**(5): 406–8.

5   Windberger U, Siegl H, Woisetschlager R *et al*. Hemodynamic changes during prolonged laparoscopic surgery. *Eur Surg Res* 1994; **26**(1): 1–9.

6   Wittgen CM, Naunheim KS, Andrus CH, Kaminski DL. Preoperative pulmonary function evaluation for laparoscopic cholecystectomy. *Arch Surg* 1993; **128**(8): 880–6.

7   Pearce DJ. Respiratory acidosis and subcutaneous emphysema during laparoscopic cholecystectomy. *Can J Anaesth* 1994; **41**(4): 314–16.

8   Schoeffler P, Bazin JE, Fourgeaud L. Anesthesia for laparoscopic surgery (in German). *Ther Umsch* 1993; **50**(8): 559–63.

9   Chin AK, Eaton J, Tsoi EK *et al*. Gasless laparoscopy using a planar lifting technique. *J Am Coll Surg* 1994; **178**(4): 401–3.

10 Smith RS, Fry WR, Tsoi EK *et al*. Gasless laparoscopy and conventional instruments. The next phase of minimally invasive surgery. *Arch Surg* 1993; **128**(10): 1102–7.

11 Volz J, Volz E, Koster S *et al*. Pelviscopic surgery without pneumoperitoneum? A new method and its effects on anesthesia (in German). *Geburtshilfe Frauenheilkd* 1993; **53**(4): 258–60.

12 Bongard FS, Pianim NA, Leighton TA *et al*. Helium insufflation for laparoscopic operation. *Surg Gynecol Obstet* 1993; **177**(2): 140–6.

13 Fitzgerald SD, Andrus CH, Baudendistel LJ, Dahms TE, Kaminski DL. Hypercarbia during carbon dioxide pneumoperitoneum. *Am J Surg* 1992; **163**(1): 186–90.

14 Andrus CH. Hemodynamic effect of argon pneumoperitoneum (comment). *Surg Endosc* 1994; **8**(4): 322–3.

15 Eisenhauer DM, Saunders CJ, Ho HS, Wolfe BM. Hemodynamic effects of argon pneumoperitoneum. *Surg Endosc* 1994; **8**(4): 315–21.

16 Prystowsky JB, Jericho BG, Epstein HM. Spontaneous bilateral pneumothorax — complication of laparoscopic cholecystectomy. *Surgery* 1993; **114**(5): 988–92.

17 Goodale RL, Beebe DS, McNevin MP *et al*. Hemodynamic, respiratory, and metabolic effects of laparoscopic cholecystectomy. *Am J Surg* 1993; **166**(5): 533–7.

18 Benhamou D, Simonneau G, Poynard T *et al*. Diaphragm function is not impaired by pneumoperitoneum after laparoscopy. *Arch Surg* 1993; **128**(4): 430–2.

19 Brampton WJ, Watson RJ. Arterial to end-tidal carbon dioxide tension difference during laparoscopy. Magnitude and effect of anaesthetic technique. *Anaesthesia* 1990; **45**(3): 210–14.

20 Safran D, Sgambati S, Orlando R. Laparoscopy in high-risk cardiac patients. *Surg Gynecol Obstet* 1993; **176**(6): 548–54.

21 Ho HS, Gunther RA, Wolfe BM. Intraperitoneal carbon dioxide insufflation and cardiopulmonary functions. Laparoscopic cholecystectomy in pigs. *Arch Surg* 1992; **127**(8): 928–33.

22 Odeberg S, Ljungqvist O, Svenberg T *et al*. Haemodynamic effects of pneumoperitoneum and the influence of posture during anaesthesia for laparoscopic surgery. *Acta Anaesth Scand* 1994; **38**(3): 276–83.

23 Moffa SM, Quinn JV, Slotman GJ. Hemodynamic effects of carbon dioxide pneumoperitoneum during mechanical ventilation and positive end-expiratory pressure. *J Trauma* 1993; **35**(4): 613–18.

24 Ishizaki Y, Bandai Y, Shimomura K *et al*. Safe intraabdominal pressure of carbon dioxide pneumoperitoneum during laparoscopic surgery. *Surgery* 1993; **114**(3) 549–54.

25 Ho HS, Saunders CJ, Corso FA, Wolfe BM. The effects of CO_2 pneumoperitoneum on hemodynamics in hemorrhaged animals. *Surgery* 1993; **114**(2): 381–8.

26 Shifren JL, Adlestein L, Finkler NJ. Asystolic cardiac arrest: a rare complication of laparoscopy. *Obstet Gynecol* 1992; **79**(5): 840–1.

27 Josephs LG, Este-McDonald JR, Birkett DH, Hirsch EF. Diagnostic laparoscopy increases intracranial pressure. *J Trauma* 1994; **36**(6): 815–19.

28 Kubota K, Kajiura N, Teruya M *et al*. Alterations in respiratory function and hemodynamics during laparoscopic cholecystectomy under pneumoperitoneum. *Surg Endosc* 1993; **7**(6): 500–4.

29 Iwase K, Takenaka H, Yagura A *et al*. Hemodynamic changes during laparoscopic cholecystectomy in patients with heart disease. *Endoscopy* 1992; **24**(9): 771–3.

30 Jorgensen JO, Lalak NJ, North L *et al*. Venous stasis during laparosocpic cholecystectomy. *Surg Laparosc Endosc* 1994; **4**(2): 128–33.

31 Millard JA, Hill BB, Cook PS, Fenoglio ME, Stahlgren LH. Intermittant sequential pneumatic compression in prevention of venous stasis associated with pneumoperitoneum during laparoscopic surgery. *Arch Surg* 1993; **128**(8): 914–19.

32 Pearson MR, Sander ML. Hyperkalaemia associated with prolonged insufflation of carbon dioxide into the peritoneal cavity. *Br J Anaesth* 1994; **72**(5): 602–4.

33 Ott DE. Laparoscopic hypothermia. *J Laparoendosc Surg* 1991a; **1**(3): 127–31.

34 Ott DE. Correction of laparoscopic insufflation hypothermia. *J Laparoendosc Surg* 1991b; **1**(4): 183–6.

35 Beck DE, McQuillan PJ. Fatal carbon dioxide embolism and severe haemorrhage during laparoscopic salpingectomy. *Br J Anaesth* 1994; **72**(2): 243–5.
36 Fredman B, Jedeikin R, Olsfanger D, Flor P, Gruzman A. Residual pneumoperitoneum: a cause of postoperative pain after laparoscopic cholecystectomy. *Anesth Analg* 1994; **79**(1): 152–4.
37 Perry CP, Tombrello R. Effect of fluid instillation on postlaparoscopy pain. *J Reprod Med* 1993; **38**(10): 768–70.

Chapter 3

Video endoscopy of the retroperitoneum

J.M. Himpens

Introduction

The first publication on retroperitoneoscopy was by Bartel in 1969 [1]. In 1976 [2] this technique was improved by Sarazin. In 1979 Hald and Rasmusen collected a series of patients, in whom staging of urological cancers had been performed by retroperitoneoscopy [3]. They used a mediastinoscope for endoscopic visualization. Wurtz [4] extended the field of retroperitoneoscopy to lumboscopy and was able to stage urological and gynaecological cancers in a minimally invasive way.

However, retroperitoneoscopy without carbon dioxide (CO_2) insufflation permitted only limited exploration of the retroperitoneum. Simple and straightforward procedures like node samplings and biopsies of retroperitoneal tumours were about all that was possible. Technical progress and the advance of powerful CO_2 insufflators and video endoscopic material markedly improved the visual and working space in the retroperitoneum. Wurtz again was the first one to introduce this technique. However, the persistence of fibrous strings which could not be taken down by CO_2 dissection limited the value of this approach.

Severance of fibrous strings can be obtained by the use of dissecting tools as proposed by Dulucq [5], Vernay and Ferzli [6]. The tediousness of this approach, however, is disappointing. In 1992, Gaur used a custom-made balloon for retroperitoneal dissection in urological procedures [7]. This technique was also used by Webb and Keizur [8], with good success. In 1994, Hirsch reported on the use of a trocar-mounted balloon dissector, permitting controlled dilatation of this preperitoneal space [9]. Balloon dissection, as well as insufflated gas, respects fascial planes, especially when no previous surgery has been performed on the site. This axioma, as explained by Meyers in 1974 [10], was confirmed by Gaur in 1992 and more recently by ourselves [11].

Unlike in laparoscopy, the abdominal wall located posteriorly is not readily distendable, and the necessary working space in retroperitoneoscopy has to be obtained by reclining the peritoneum to condense the internal organs and thus create a working space.

As the fascial planes are respected by balloon dissection, perfect knowledge of the anatomy and, more specifically, of the sometimes subtle fasciae is mandatory for the surgeon involved in retroperitoneoscopy.

Anatomy

Retropubic space

The most important structure in the retropubic or Retzius space is the bladder. Because of its distendibility, and the fact that the peritoneum reflects only on its anterosuperior part, the space of Retzius is easily accessible for balloon dilatation. The bladder is covered by a fascia, containing the urachus in the midline, which constitutes the median umbilical vault. Laterally this fascia contains fibrous strands, remnants of the degenerated umbilical arteries, and constitutes the medial umbilical vault. These vaults overlie the inferior epigastric vessels. At that level the fascia is very adherent to the epigastrics. This adherent area constitutes the frontier line between the Retzius space medially and the Bogros space laterally. Balloon dilatation of the Retzius space will usually respect the fascial adhesions at the level of the epigastrics and will not, therefore, permit direct access to the Bogros space out of the Retzius.

The anterior wall of the Retzius space is the bare abdominal wall. This wall, constituted at this level by the rectus muscle, is covered deeply by the fascia transversalis. This transversalis fascia blends more cranially into the posterior rectus sheath. The fusion of fascia with this sheath occurs at the level of the arcade of Douglas.

In conclusion, the boundaries of the Retzius space — the true retropubic retroperitoneum — are: (i) anteriorly the pubis with, cranially to it, the transversalis fascia as described by Cooper [12], and more cranially blending into the posterior rectus sheath; (ii) laterally the epigastric vessels adherent with expansions of the prevesical fascia; and (iii) dorsally the bladder covered by prevesical fascia containing the median and medial umbilical ligaments. This prevesical fascia is a condensation of the peritoneum, but could also be an extension of the transversalis fascia [13,14].

Iliac retroperitoneum

The lateral suprainguinal space of Bogros [15] is located laterally to the epigastrics, deep to the anterior abdominal wall and limited by the pelvic wall laterally. The floor of the Bogros space is the psoas muscle, carrying medially to it the iliac vessels and the femoral nerve. The Bogros space or iliac retroperitoneum lies in direct continuity with the lumbar retroperitoneum. Direct insufflation of the Bogros space can be obtained by insertion of a balloon through the anterior abdominal wall, lateral to the epigastrics and cranial to the internal inguinal ring. This is basically the approach described by McEvedy-Nyhus [16].

Lumbar retroperitoneum

Central to the anatomy of the lumbar retroperitoneum is the kidney. The kidney is enveloped by the fascia (Gerota's fascia), which envelopes the kidney, adrenal gland and perirenal fat (Fig. 3.1).

This fascia has the shape of a cone, is closed cranially, is adherent to the diaphragm on the left and the liver on the right, is open distally, and is in free communication with Bogros' space. Laterally, Gerota's fascia is connected with the lateroposterior parietal peritoneum, in close relationship with the ascending colon on the right and the descending colon on the left. This lateral expansion of

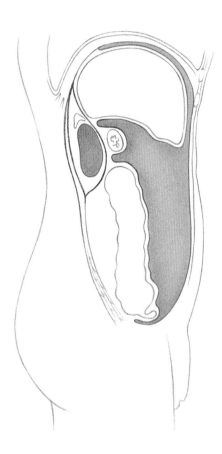

Figure 3.1
Sagittal section at the level of the ® anterior axillary line.

Gerota's fascia is called the lateroconal fascia [10] and separates the lumbar retroperitoneum into an anterior pararenal space, medial to the lateroconal fascia and anterior to the anterior Gerota's fascia, and a posterior pararenal space located laterally to the lateroconal fascia and dorsally to the posterior aspect of Gerota's fascia (Fig. 3.2).

Medially, the Gerota fascia opens to permit the entrance of the vascular pedicle to the kidney. The anterior aspect of Gerota's fascia therefore covers the vena cava and the aorta. The posterior layer of Gerota's fascia fuses with the fascia overlying the psoas muscle. This band of fusion is located over the belly of the psoas muscle and, therefore, the posterior pararenal space is not in continuity with the medial border of the psoas muscle. This is the reason why the fascia has to be perforated if one wants to reach the sympathetic chain through the posterior pararenal space [17].

In conclusion, the pararenal space is divided into an anterior and a posterior pararenal space, with its limit being marked by the lateroconal fascia.

Since Gerota's fascia is a cone open distally and ending rather abruptly, the iliac retroperitoneum distal to this cone will be in free connection with the anterior and posterior pararenal spaces and the entire perirenal space. If a balloon is inserted into the iliac retroperitoneum (Fig. 3.3) distally to the perirenal fascia, a working space can be obtained from where the two pararenal spaces and the perirenal space can be entered. Since the mass of the kidney is usually sizeable and there is perirenal fat accumulated within Gerota's fascia, dissection around this mass is prone to confusion.

The best landmark available in this area is the lateroconal fascia. This fascia is situated in the sagittal plane, uniting the lateral aspect of Gerota's fascia with the

Figure 3.2
Cross-section of the body showing the posterior pararenal space 'at rest'.

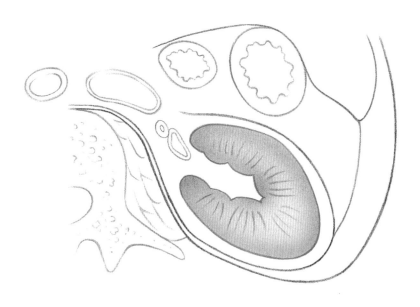

Figure 3.3
Cross-section showing the posterior pararenal space and the changes caused by balloon insufflation.

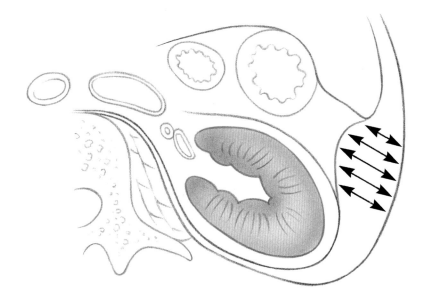

posterolateral aspect of the parietal peritoneum, and overlying the colon. If a balloon is inflated dorsally and laterally to the kidney, balloon compression will give this lateroconal fascia the appearance of a semicylinder with its concavity facing the posterolateral abdominal wall (Fig. 3.4). Since this fascia, as well as Gerota's fascia, ends very abruptly distally it will present a free distal edge running anteroposteriorly and in continuity with the distal edge of the posterior pararenal fascia, inserting on the ventral aspect of the psoas muscle and fascia.

Incision of the lateroconal fascia, starting midway at its free edge and expanding cranially, obviously opens up the anterior pararenal space. The contents of the space that are easily in reach from this approach are the descending part of the duodenum on the right and, more medially, the head of the pancreas. The vena cava cannot be reached from this approach as Gerota's

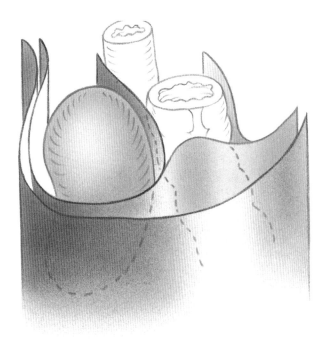

Figure 3.4
Lateral view of the pararenal space after balloon insufflation. Note the displacement of the lateroconal fascia.

fascia covers its anterior aspect. The anterior pararenal space contains, on the left, the tail of the pancreas and the splenic vessels. Again, and for the same reason as for the vena cava, the aorta can not be reached via the anterior pararenal space because of the overlying anterior perirenal fascia.

If one elects to dissect the vena cava (on the right) or the aorta (on the left), one has to start dissecting distally and medially to the lateroconal fascia. No fascia layers have to be incised if one departs from the iliac fossa and stays between the anterior and posterior Gerota's fascia; this makes the abdominal vessels reachable medially.

Localizing the lateroconal fascia therefore constitutes the most important step in extrarenal retroperitoneoscopic work. It also guarantees the integrity of the peritoneum which is very easily torn in the high lumbar space.

Instruments

Retroperitoneoscopy demands specific instrumentation. The necessary working space is obtained by the insufflation of a balloon (PDB balloon, Origin Medsystems, Menlo Park, California, USA). The advantage of this type of balloon is that the laparoscope can be placed inside while insufflating and one can therefore be sure about expanding the correct space. After insufflation, the balloon trocar is replaced by an air-sealing trocar (Blunt tip, Origin Medsystems). Additional trocars (usually three) are inserted under direct vision. They allow the insertion of a coagulating hook, a grasping forceps, a peanut dissector and an automatic clip applier. The hand-like retractor (Endoretract, USSC, Norwalk, Connecticut, USA) has proven very useful in reclining the peritoneum, especially in high retroperitoneoscopy. Ligation of vessels is obtained by clips or by suture ligation. Knots can be tied either intracorporeally or extracorporeally.

Surgical technique

Retropubic retroperitoneoscopy

In this procedure the operative field is limited to the Retzius space. An incision is made infraumbilically, just off the midline. The dissection is carried down to the anterior rectus sheath, the sheath is grasped with two forceps and is incised. The rectus muscle fibres are reclined laterally until the posterior rectus sheath is reached. The balloon trocar is inserted and pushed down to the pubis. It is then insufflated under direct vision. The epigastrics should be seen on both sides and it is imperative that they stay in contact with the abdominal wall. This goal is usually achieved by pushing the balloon trocar dorsally while inflating. After a good working space has been obtained, two trocars are placed just medial to the epigastrics, about half way between the pubis and umbilicus.

In a Burch procedure the retropubic space is dissected on both sides of the urethra. The endopelvic fascia (obturator fascia) is clearly visualized. By doing this dissection the bladder is pushed cranially, hereby exposing the anterior wall of the vagina. The anchoring of the anterior vaginal wall to Cooper's ligament is usually straightforward.

In obturator nodal sampling the triangle between the iliac vein, obturator nerve and pubis and obturator fascia is completely cleared with a grasper and a coagulating hook. The nodal samples are usually easily delivered through the trocars.

Iliac retroperitoneoscopy

The initial approach to iliac retroperitoneoscopy is the same as for retropubic retroperitoneoscopy. After balloon dilatation, however, only one working trocar is inserted. It is placed off the midline, on the opposite side of the dissected area, half way between the pubis and umbilicus. A peanut dissector is used and is gently inserted in the space between the epigastrics and the spermatic cord (or round ligament). As described above, the peritoneum is very adherent to the epigastrics in this area. Once the space between the epigastrics and the spermatic cord is opened, the Bogros space is reached. The peritoneum is now easily brushed away from the psoas muscle.

In cases of a low appendectomy scar, the peritoneum can be very firmly stuck to the abdominal wall. It is better to avoid these adhesions by contouring them, rather than risking an accidental tear in the peritoneum at this stage which might jeopardize further dissection.

In patients with a hernia, one additional trocar is inserted just cephalad to the superior and anterior iliac spine. For other procedures, where the aim of dissection is located more medially, two additional working trocars are inserted in the right lower quadrant under direct vision. The endoscope is replaced in one of the right lower quadrant trocars.

The subumbilical sealing trocar will usually contain the hand-like retractor (USSC) and dissection is carried out bimanually, according to the triangulation principle. Medially located structures (ureter, sympathetic chain and para-aortic nodes) can easily be visualized and dissected with this technique.

Lumbar retroperitoneoscopy

As mentioned above, the most important landmark in the high retroperitoneum is the kidney. The kidney itself, surrounded by fat, is protected by the perirenal (Gerota) fascia. The anterior sheath of this fascia fuses with the periadventitial tissue of the vena cava and aorta. Its posterior sheath reaches the ventral aspect of the psoas muscle medially. Laterally, the perirenal fascia is connected with the peritoneum by the lateroconal fascia located in a sagittal plane.

If the aim of the dissection is to reach the duodenum, the head of the pancreas on the right or the tail of the pancreas on the left, the lateroconal fascia is the landmark of choice. If a balloon is inflated laterally in the posterior pararenal space, which is the easiest to reach, the lateroconal fascia is condensed and insinuates itself in the space between the kidney posteriorly and the colon anteriorly. Therefore, the anterior pararenal space is best reached by the following procedure.

1 Performing an iliac retroperitoneoscopy.
2 Inflating a balloon in the lateral posterior pararenal space, under direct vision, and keeping the balloon aimed anteriorly.
3 Inserting three working trocars, one on the midclavicular and two on the anterior axillary line, on both sides of the midclavicular line.
4 Reclining the peritoneal sac away from the kidney, through the midclavicular trocar. This will put the lateroconal fascia under traction.
5 Dividing the lateroconal fascia longitudinally in its deepest recess.
6 Dissecting the loose areolar tissue deep to this fascia until the anterior pararenal space opens up.

If the target, however, is the kidney or the adrenals it is essential not to violate the lateroconal fascia. The easiest way to avoid this in the author's opinion is to locate the ureter and follow it upwards. This will bring the surgeon into the right plane within the Gerota fascia, which is very suitable for kidney surgery. For the adrenals, however, performing an iliac retroperitoneoscopy demands a lot more dissection before the target organ is reached. It is probably better to centre the dissection by entering the retroperitoneum at a higher level. An interesting approach has been described by Mercan [18] who uses a retroperitoneal route with the patient in the prone position, hereby confirming the experimental work of several authors. The initial incision is performed over the kidney (ultrasound or fluoroscopy [19] can be helpful). Once the kidney surface is reached by finger dissection, the balloon trocar is inserted and inflated. The entire perirenal space is insufflated creating a very acceptable working space [18], and working trocars are then inserted under direct vision and the adrenal dissected. The coagulating hook is the most suitable tool in the author's opinion to perform this dissection.

Future perspectives

An exciting new area of development could be vascular work undertaken via the laparoscopic approach. Dion *et al.* [20] first described a laparoscopically assisted aortobifemoral bypass. Dulucq [21] performed the first aortoiliacal bypass laparoscopically (J.L. Dulucq, personal communication). The development of retroperitoneoscopic techniques will soon render the videoscopic approach suitable for classic retroperitoneal work.

References

1 Bartel M. Die Retroperitoneoskopie. Eine endoskopische methode zur inspektion und bioptischen untersuchung des retroperitonealen. *Zentralbl Chir* 1969; **94**: 377–83.
2 Vernay A. La rétropéritonéoscopie: justification anatomique. Expérimentation technique. Expérience clinique. PhD thesis, Grenoble, 1980.
3 Hald T, Rasmussen F. Extraperitoneal pelvioscopy: a new aid in staging of lower urinary tract tumors. A preliminary report. *J Urol* 1980; **124**: 245–8.
4 Wurtz A. L'endoscopie de l'espace rétropéritonéal: techniques, résultats et indications actuelles. *Ann Chir* 1989; **43**: 475–80.
5 Dulucq JL. Traitement des hernies de l'aine par mise en place d'un patch prothétique sous-péritonéal en rétropéritonéoscopie. *Cah Chirurg* 1991; **79**: 15–16.
6 Ferzli G, Raboy A, Kleinerman D, Albert P. Extraperitoneal endoscopic pelvic lymph node dissection vs laparoscopic lymph node dissection in the staging of prostatic and bladder carcinoma. *J Laparoendosc Surg* 1992; **2**: 219–22.
7 Gaur DD. Laparoscopic operative retroperitoneoscopy: use of a new device. *J Urol* 1992; **148**: 1137–9.
8 Webb DR, Redgrave N, Chan Y, Harewood LM. Extraperitoneal laparoscopy: early experience and evaluation. *Aust N Z J Surg* 1993; **63**: 554–7.
9 Hirsch IH, Morena JG, Lotfi MA, Ch MBB, Gomella LG. Controlled balloon dilatation of the extraperitoneal space for laparoscopic urologic surgery. *J Laparoendosc Surg* 1994; **4**(4): 247–51.
10 Meyers MA. The spread and localization of acute intraperitoneal effusions. *Radiology* 1970; **95**: 547–54.
11 Himpens J, Van Alphen P, Cadière GB, Verroken R. Balloon dissection in extended retroperitoneoscopy. *Surg Laparosc Endosc* 1994; **5**: 193–6.
12 Cooper PA. *The Anatomy and Surgical Treatment of Abdominal Hernia*, Parts 1 and 2. London: Longman, 1804–1807.
13 Read RC. Cooper's posterior lamina of transversalis fascia. *Surg Gynecol Obstet* 1992; **174**: 426.
14 Lampe EW. Special comment: transversalis fascia. In: Nyhus LM, Condon RE (eds) *Hernia*, 2nd edn. Philadelphia: JB Lippincott, 1978: 60.
15 Bogros AJ. Essai sur l'anatomie chirurgicales de la region iliaque et desciption d'un nouveau procédé pour faire la ligature des artères épigastrique et iliaque externe. Th Paris 1823, no. 153. Paris, Didot le Jeune rue des Macons, Sorbonne no. 13.
16 McVay CB, Read RC, Ravitch MM. Inguinal hernia. *Curr Probl Surg* 1964; 10.
17 Madden JL. Left lumbar sympathetic ganglionectomy. In: Madden JL (ed.). *Atlas and Technique in Surgery*, 2nd edn. New York: Appleton-Century Crofts, 1958: 100.
18 Mercan S. Videoscopic retroperitoneal adrenalectomy. Communication: general surgery motion picture session. Presented to the American College of Surgeons, 80th Annual Congress, Chicago, October 1994.
19 Brunt LM, Molmenti EP, Kebl K *et al*. Retroperitoneal endoscopic adrenalectomy an experimental study. *Surg Laparosc Endosc* 1993; **3**(4): 300–6.
20 Dion YM, Katkhouda N, Rouleau CL, Aucoin A. Laparoscopy-assisted aortobifemoral bypass. *Surg Laparosc Endosc* 1993; **3**: 425–9.

Chapter 4

Retroperitoneal colonic mobilization

R.J. Stacey and A.W. Darzi

Introduction

Laparoscopic colonic surgery has not developed at the same pace as other laparoscopic procedures because of the requirement for advanced skills in laparoscopic surgery and concerns regarding the technique. In particular these include increased operating time, risk of damage to vital retroperitoneal structures and concerns that laparoscopic resections may not be adequate for neoplasia.

Although the colon is a retroperitoneal structure, in most descriptions of colonic mobilization, either laparoscopic or open, colectomy is performed via a transperitoneal route. In this chapter we describe a combined technique involving both laparoscopic and retroperitoneoscopic approaches to colonic mobilization using specifically designed balloons and operating in the retroperitoneal space.

Surgical technique

Full video endoscopic facilities are required including the provision of a camera, television monitor and insufflation system for both laparoscopy and retroperitoneoscopy (Fig. 4.1).

Laparoscopy

Standard preoperative preparations are employed including anti-thrombotic measures, routine bowel preparation and antibiotic prophylaxis. A nasogastric tube and urinary catheter are passed after anaesthesia and the patient is positioned in a modified Lloyd-Davies position with minimal hip flexion. A pneumoperitoneum is established using a standard method for insufflation with a Veress needle, and is maintained at 12–16 mmHg by an automatic carbon dioxide (CO_2) insufflator. A 10 mm 0° laparoscope is inserted through a subumbilical port and initial laparoscopy is performed. At this stage the feasibility of resection is assessed.

Retroperitoneoscopy

A 2 cm incision is made just above the anterior superior iliac spine and the subcutaneous and fascial layers are dissected down to the iliacus and quadratus

Figure 4.1
Theatre set-up with both laparoscopy and retroperitoneoscopy.

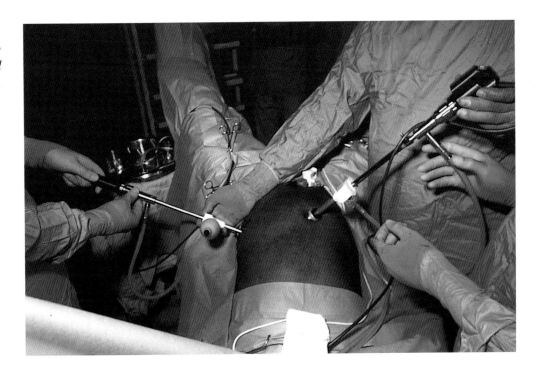

lumborum muscles. Continuous laparoscopic monitoring ensures that the peritoneum is not violated. A modified preperitoneal latex balloon is then inserted into the retroperitoneal space behind either the ascending or descending colon depending on operation site (Fig. 4.2). At this stage, the laparoscope is passed through the retroperitoneal 'balloon' port (Fig. 4.3) and gentle dissection is commenced by distending the balloon with a hand-held bulb insufflator. The transparent balloon surrounds the retroperitoneal laparoscope allowing direct visualization of the vital retroperitoneal structures during distension, including the ureter, gonadal vessels and, on the right side, the duodenum.

Figure 4.2
Retroperitoneal balloon distension resulting in colonic mobilization.

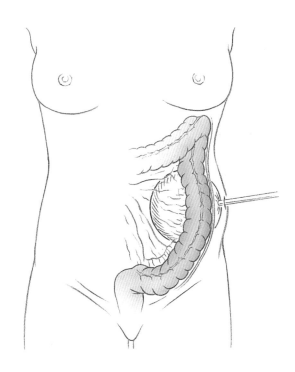

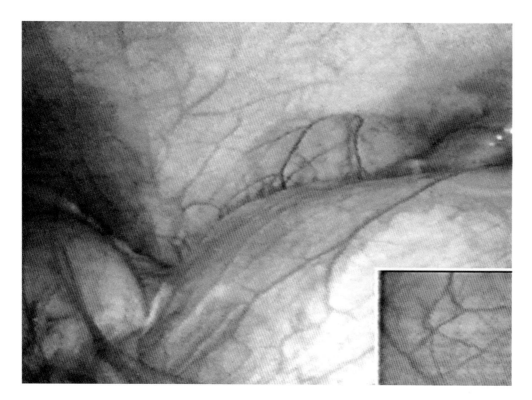

Figure 4.3
Laparoscopic view of retroperitoneal balloon distension; the insert shows the view from the retroperitoneal camera.

The retroperitoneal distension process is simultaneously monitored by a second laparoscope inserted through the umbilicus. Careful balloon distension is used initially to create a small lateral space into which CO_2 may be introduced for further dissection. This avoids the possibility of trapping the ureter and gonadal vessels against the posterior abdominal wall. After initial mobilization the balloon port is replaced by a 10 mm occlusion port and the cavity thus formed is distended with CO_2. The retroperitoneal endoscope is passed through the retroperitoneal port and, under direct vision, two further 5 mm ports are inserted. This allows the introduction of grasping forceps which are used to carefully peel off any structures which are adherent to the undersurface of the peritoneum (Fig. 4.4). In this way vital structures are identified and gently placed against the posterior abdominal wall well away from the now mobilized peritoneum.

As dissection proceeds, the colonic mesentery is elevated and particularly good views are obtained of the aortic origins of the vascular pedicle (Fig. 4.5). This allows flush ligation, under direct vision, using the Endo-GIA (Autosutre, Ascot, UK) stapling device. When this has been achieved complete and accurate excision of the lymphatic drainage field is now possible. Once mobilization is complete, two further intraperitoneal ports are inserted under direct vision in the contralateral hypochondrium and iliac fossa for the use of laparoscopic hooked scissors and graspers.

Standard laparoscopically assisted colectomy involves bowel retraction, mobilization, division of mesenteric vessels and delivery of the bowel to the skin surface for resection and subsequent anastomosis [1,2]. Using the retroperitoneal approach, colonic mobilization is almost complete except for the division of the peritoneal reflection (Fig. 4.6). With the retroperitoneal space distended with CO_2 the colonic peritoneal reflection is divided accurately with scissors, operating from the laparoscopic ports, without risk to retroperitoneal structures (Fig. 4.7).

Figure 4.4
The view via the retroperitoneal camera once distension is complete showing the psoas muscle, the ureter and gonadal vessels.

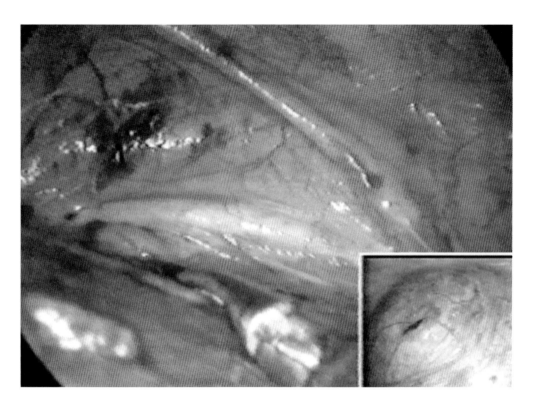

Figure 4.5
The inferior mesenteric vessels mobilized to their origin.

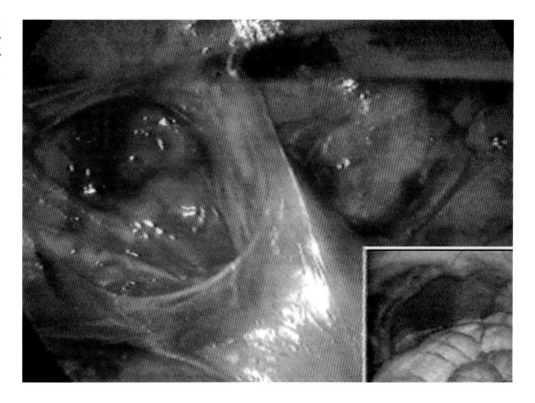

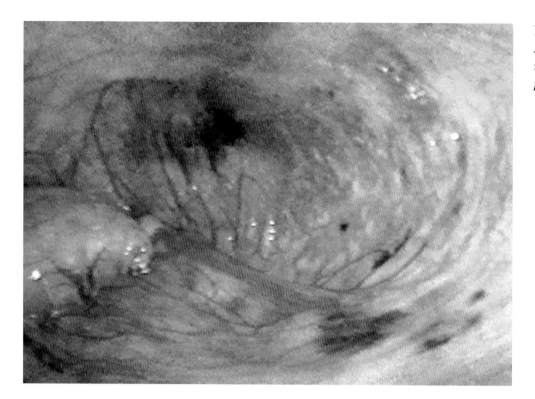

Figure 4.6
A laparoscopic view of the mobilized colon with the peritoneal reflection intact.

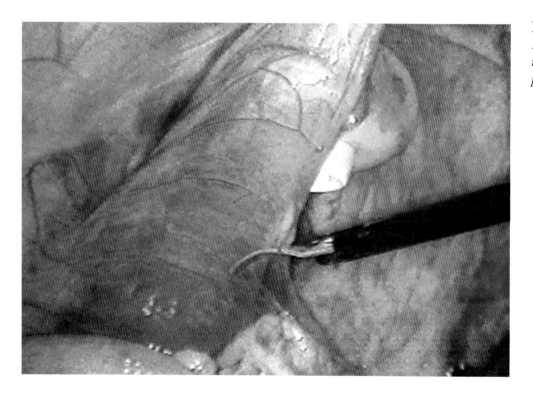

Figure 4.7
Division of the peritoneal reflection via the laparoscopic ports.

High mesenteric vascular ligation has already been performed and the relevant bowel section, thus mobilized, is delivered through a small skin incision for resection and anastomosis. Thus far this method of colonic mobilization has been performed successfully, via an open laparotomy wound and as a fully laparoscopic procedure in patients with full informed consent [3].

Discussion

Laparoscopic colonic surgery has the same potential benefits of decreased postoperative pain and shorter postoperative stay associated with laparoscopic cholecystectomy [4]. The technique has, however, been criticised with doubts over oncological safety, increased operating time and problems with accurate identification and preservation of vital retroperitoneal structures [5,6]. With the use of retroperitoneoscopy and balloon-assisted blunt colonic mobilization, the potential for sharp or diathermy-related injuries and overall operating time is reduced. This technique also provides particularly clear views of the mesenteric vessels allowing division at their origin and thus complete excision of the lymphatic drainage field. Colonic mobilization, whether open or laparoscopic, is traditionally performed by sharp division of the peritoneal reflection. This is followed by blunt mobilization of the colon and its mesentery off the retroperitoneal structures [7]. In laparoscopic colonic mobilization, retraction of the colon at two fixed points is essential to achieve adequate tension on the peritoneal reflection. This has the disadvantage of adding extra ports and also requiring the use of Babcock-type grasping forceps which might traumatize the bowel. In our experience the time required to achieve adequate colonic mobilization is shorter when employing balloon dissectors. Similar balloon dissectors are now being employed in extraperitoneal hernia repair and most reports suggest that this technique facilitates and shortens the operating time.

Retroperitoneoscopy is an exciting new approach in endoscopic surgery. Recent reports of the extraperitoneal technique in hernia repair, nephrectomy, lumbar sympathectomy and even adrenalectomy [8] has revolutionized this approach to retroperitoneal structures. The colon and rectum, with the exception of the transverse colon, are retroperitoneal structures and we feel that retroperitoneoscopy and balloon dilatation have unique advantages, especially in identifying vital retroperitoneal structures early in the procedure. It is obvious that caution should be employed when dealing with colonic neoplasia. If the initial laparoscopy suggests that the tumour is fixed, the authors feel that an open approach is best adopted.

References

1   Darzi A, Hill ADK, Henry MM, Guillou PJ, Monson JRT. Laparoscopic surgery of the colon — operative technique. *Endosc Surg Allied Technol* 1993; **1**: 13–15.
2   Fowler DL, White SA. Laparoscopic assisted sigmoid resection. *Surg Laparosc Endosc* 1991; **1**(3): 283–8.
3   Darzi AW, Hunt N, Stacey RJ. Retroperitoneoscopy and retroperitoneal colonic mobilization: a new approach in laparoscopic colonic surgery. *Br J Surg* 1995; **82**: 1038–9
4   Southern Surgeons Club. A prospective analysis of 1518 laparoscopic cholecystectomies. *N Engl J Med* 1991; **324**: 1073–8.

5   Guillou PJ, Darzi A, Monson JRT. Experience with laparoscopic colorectal surgery for malignant disease. *Surg Oncol* 1993; **2**(Suppl): 43–9.

6   Warshaw AL. Reflections on laparoscopic surgery (editorial). *Surgery* 1993; **114**: 629–30.

7   Monson JRT, Darzi A, Carey PD, Guillou PJ. Prospective evaluation of laparoscopic assisted colectomy in an unselected group of patients. *Lancet* 1992; **340**: 831–3.

8   Brunt LM, Molmenti EP, Kerbl K, Stone MS, Clayman RV. Retroperitoneal endoscopic adrenalectomy: an experimental study. *Surg Laparosc Endosc* 1993; **3**: 300–6.

Chapter 5
Endoscopic extraperitoneal lumbar sympathectomy

P. Hourlay

Introduction

The first lumbar sympathectomy was performed in 1923 by Dr D. Royle in Sydney for the treatment of unilateral spastic paralysis of the leg [1,2]. The postoperative evaluation showed side effects of local warmth and capillary vasodilation. For this reason lumbar sympathectomy was also performed for thromboangitis obliterans and later on a more regular basis for vascular problems of the leg [2,3]. A sympathectomy not only causes a relaxation of the arteriovenous anastomoses, explaining the vasodilation of the skin, but also causes an interruption of the pain-afferent pathways. Therefore, Sudeck atrophy is an indication for sympathectomy.

The possibility of performing a sympathectomy as a minimally invasive surgical technique will probably increase the indications of the procedure. Until recently limited to the treatment of peripheral endstage vascular diseases with cutaneous ischaemia, the lumbar sympathectomy performed by this new type of approach can be indicated in cases of hyperhydrosis and for pain treatment (neuroalgodystrophy).

Surgical technique

The procedure is performed under general anaesthesia when using carbon dioxide (CO_2) to maintain the working space. The use of low pressure CO_2 insufflation and endoscopic mechanical retractors allows the procedure to be done under regional or local anaesthesia (which is more technically demanding). The installation of the patient is identical to the installation for a kidney intervention — that is with the patient in a lumbotomy position, 45° laterally. The table is broken at level L3 (Fig 5.1). The installation provides the surgeon with a good exposition for the endoscopic procedure and allows the possibility of access to the peritoneal cavity if needed.

Extraperitoneal blunt dissection between the muscle and peritoneum is started with the finger through a 12 mm MacBurney incision. This blunt dissection progresses laterally in the direction of the psoas muscle. A very elegant alternative technique for entering the extraperitoneal space consists of using a transparent and cutting trocar (Visiport, USSC, Norwalk, Connecticut, USA). Although this trocar has been created for penetrating into the peritoneal cavity after previous surgery (with possible adhesions) under view control after CO_2

Figure 5.1
Position of the patient on the table.

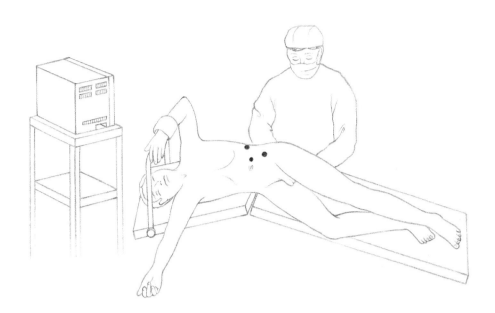

insufflation, it is used in extraperitoneal surgery to begin the creation of the extraperitoneal working space. It is introduced through a 11 mm surgical incision (the right or left MacBurney region). The anterior fascia is cut and the muscle layer is split by pushing on the instrument. The CO_2 insufflation transforms the virtual space between the muscles and peritoneal membrane into a real working space. This manoeuvre, carefully done under view control, allows a fast and safe creation of an extraperitoneal space through a limited skin incision. A purse-string suture is placed through the skin and subcutaneous tissue to avoid CO_2 leakage during insufflation.

A first trocar (the blunt port or trocar of the transparent and cutting device) is inserted through the small incision (Fig 5.2). A correct placement of the trocar in the extraperitoneal space between the peritoneum and muscles is checked with the camera. The purse-string suture is closed round the trocar and CO_2 is insufflated. The flow of CO_2 varies from 2 to 10 l/min.

Extraperitoneal blunt dissection is continued under visual control, using the scope as a blunt dissector (Fig. 5.3). This scope dissection is performed in the direction of the spinal column, to the medial side of the psoas, following the line of the psoas muscle. In this way, the extraperitoneal cavity is progressively created. Turning the patient on to the controlateral side is helpful (Fig. 5.4). A second 11 mm port is inserted under visual control at the junction of the lumbar region and the flank, at the level of the umbilicus. The scope is then transferred into this trocar.

A specially designed 10 mm dissector is introduced through the first trocar. This allows the dissection to be continued along the abdominal aorta or vena cava and vertebrae. A 5 mm port is placed under visual control at level L3–L2 in the umbilical region, at the medial limit of the extraperitoneal dissection. An atraumatic grasper and shears with monopolar coagulation are introduced through the first and third trocars. The sympathetic chain lies inside the insertions of the psoas muscle.

A gauze swab held by the grasper is used to clearly visualize the sympathetic chain. The magnification of the laparoscope provides the surgeon with a very

Figure 5.2
Trocar placement (front view).

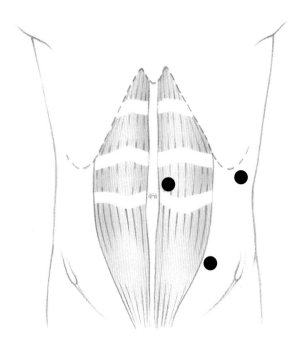

Figure 5.3
Front view of the route from the initial incision up to the sympathetic chain.

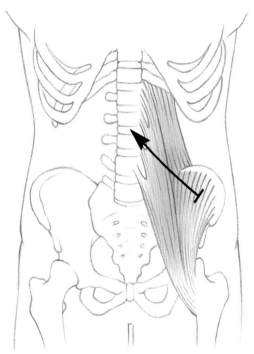

accurate identification of the anatomical structures. A segment of nerve fibres, including the L3–L2 ganglions, is resected. During this dissection, great care must be taken in order not to traumatize the iliac vessels, ureter and spermatic vessels. Bleeding of a lumbar vessel is controlled by compression and/or clip placement.

A perforation of the peritoneum reduces the extraperitoneal working space. It is possible to avoid this complication by using specially designed blunt dissectors developed to create the extraperitoneal cavity. If a perforation in the peritoneum should occur, a Veress needle is inserted in the peritoneal cavity in order to

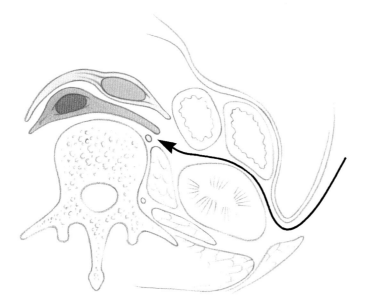

evacuate the intraperitoneal CO_2. The tension-free peritoneal membrane can then be closed using a clip applier.

A drain can be placed in the extraperitoneal cavity and this catheter is usually removed 24 hours postoperatively.

The pitfalls (Table 5.1) and tricks (Table 5.2) of extraperitoneal surgical endoscopy must be known in order to increase the feasibility of the procedure and avoid the preoperative complications.

Other methods of trocar installation have been described where the dissection is not started distally and the area of the abdomen where the trocars are placed is smaller. The installation described in this chapter results in a better divergence of the laparoscopic instrumentation. Following the psoas muscle to the sympathetic chain means that the procedure can be reproduced. This approach is also suitable for reaching the big abdominal vessels, the ureter (from the bladder up to the kidney) and the kidney. The progressive creation of the extraperitoneal space makes the procedure feasible for patients who have undergone previous extraperitoneal surgery.

- Gas leakage around the first trocar (purse-string suture or fixation system not adequate)
- False dissection plan
- Small working space available when there is:
  difficulty of retraction of intra- or extra-abdominal organs
  bad positioning of the ports
- Working space lost when there is:
  bad muscle relaxation
  bleeding
  perforation of the peritoneum
  gas leakage around the working trocars
- Excessive CO_2 resorption
- Subcutaneous emphysema
- Trauma to important anatomical structures

Table 5.1
Pitfalls of extraperitoneal endoscopy.

Table 5.2
Tricks of extraperitoneal endoscopy.

- Perfect access technique
- Checking:
  the position of the first trocar before tightening the purse-string suture
  that the first trocar is hermetically sealed
- The whole dissection and each manoeuvre is under visual control
- Understanding the importance of the patient's position and the table movements
- Insertion of working trocars at the external boundary of the created space
- Maximal muscle relaxation during the whole procedure
- Careful haemostasis and swabbing in the working space
- Blunt atraumatic dissectors
- Closure of the peritoneum openings (using a lower extraperitoneal CO_2 flow and an intraperitoneal Veress needle)
- Adaptation of gas pressure and flow
- Specific atraumatic autostatic retractor
- Lens with an incorporated cleaning channel or with an external lens cleaner

Clinical experience

The author has operated on 14 patients for endoscopic lumbar sympathectomy. Twelve patients suffered from Sudeck atrophy and two patients presented with a peripheral endstage vascular disease with cutaneous ischaemia. Eleven left-sided and three right-sided sympathectomies were performed. One of these patients presented with a previous nephrectomy and an unsuccessful previous open sympathectomy on the same side. The mean operating time was 38 minutes and the postoperative hospital stay was 2 days. In all cases, the clinical result was identical to that achieved with an open sympathectomy. No preoperative complications have been noted.

In the author's opinion this new extraperitoneal endoscopic approach for lumbar sympathectomy is as safe and as efficient as the open procedure, and also offers the advantages of minimally invasive surgery. The totally extraperitoneal approach avoids intraperitoneal manoeuvres and their possible consequences — laparoscopy-related complications, postoperative adhesions and shoulder pain.

References

1   Janoff KA, Phinney ES, Porter JM. Lumbar sympathectomy for lower extremity vasospasm. *Am J Surg* 1985; **150**(1): 146–52.
2   Kissling R, Sager M. Morbus Sudeck — Erscheinungsbild und Therapie. *Unfallchirugie* 1990; **16**: 88–94 (Nr 2).
3   Persson AV. Selection of patients for lumbar sympathectomy. *Surg Clin North Am* 1985; **65**: 2.

Further reading

AbuRahma AF, Robinson PA. Clinical parameters for predicting response to lumbar sympathectomy in patients with severe lower limb ischemia. *J Cardiovasc Surg* 1990; **31**: 101–6.
Cotton LT, Cross FW. Lumbar sympathectomy for arterial disease. *Br J Surg* 1985; **72**: 678–83.
Ellis H. Lumbar sympathectomy. *Br J Hosp Med* 1986; **35**: 124–5.
Haraway RA. The treatment of chronic extremity pain in failed lumbar surgery: the role of lumbar sympathectomy. *Spine* 1993; **18**(15): 2367–8.
Hourlay P, Vangertruyden G, Verduyckt F, Trimpeneers F, Hendrickx J. Endoscopic extraperitoneal lumbar sympathectomy. *Surg Endosc* 1995; **9**: 530–3.

Kruse CA. Thirty year experience with predictive lumbar sympathectomy. Method for selection of patients. *Am J Surg* 1985; **150**(2): 232–6.

Massell TB. Causalgic form of postphlebitic syndrome. A variety of reflex sympathetic dystrophy caused by acute deep thrombophlebitis. *West J Med* 1988; **149**(8): 294–5.

Mockus MB, Rutherford RB, Rosales C, Pearce WH. Sympathectomy for causalgia. *Arch Surg* 1987; **122**: 668–72.

Moran KT, Brady MF. Surgical management of primary hyperhydrosis. *Br J Surg* 1991; **78**(3): 279–83.

Norman PE, House AK. The early use of operative lumbar sympathectomy in peripheral vascular disease. *J Cardiovasc Surg* 1988; **29**: 492–5.

Olcott C IV, Eltherington LG, Wilcosky BR, Shoor PM, Zimmerman JJ, Fogarthy TJ. Reflex sympathetic dystrophy — the surgeon's role in management. *J Vasc Surg* 1991; **14**(4): 488–92; discussion 492–5.

Petriccione di Vadi P, Hamann W. Continuous lumbar sympathetic block. *Clin J Pain* 1991; **7**(3): 230–1.

Repelear van Driel OJ, van Bockel JH, van Schilfgaarde R. Lumbar sympathectomy for severe lower limb ischemia: results and analysis of factors influencing the outcome. *J Cardiovasc Surg* 1988; **29**: 310–14.

Rivers SP, Veith FJ, Ascer E, Gupta SK. Successful conservative therapy of severe limb-threatening ischemia: the value of non-sympathectomy. *Surgery* 1986; **99**(6): 759–62.

Vulpio C, Borzone A, Iannace C *et al*. Lumbar chemic sympathectomy in end stage of arterial disease: early and late results. *Angiology* 1989; **40**(11): 948–52.

Wang JK, Johnson KA, Ilstrug DM. Sympathetic blocks for reflex sympathetic dystrophy. *Pain* 1985; **23**: 13–17.

Chapter 6
Retroperitoneoscopy and nephrectomy

D.D. Gaur

Introduction

The historical report of a laparoscopic nephrectomy performed transperitoneally by Clayman *et al.* in 1991 [1], aroused a worldwide interest in laparoscopic surgery of the retroperitoneal organs. Clayman *et al.* even performed a retroperitoneal laparoscopic nephrectomy but, as they found the technique unsatisfactory, their subsequent nephrectomies were mostly performed transperitoneally [2]. It was only after the author reported the first case of retroperitoneal laparoscopic nephrectomy [3] using his balloon technique [4] that there was a sudden increase in the number of retroperitoneal laparoscopic procedures undertaken [5–20].

The conventional technique of retroperitoneoscopy involved the creation of a pneumoretroperitoneum simply by insufflation through a Veress needle placed percutaneously in the retroperitoneal space. This was mostly unsuccessful as the tough fibrofatty and areola tissue present in the retroperitoneum [21] does not permit the creation of a satisfactory pneumoretroperitoneum without prior mechanical dissection. The author's balloon technique of retroperitoneoscopy solved the problem as it created a space in the retroperitoneum by breaking down the fibroareolar septae. The balloon also neatly and atraumatically dissects the retroperitoneal organs, compresses the loose fibrofatty and areolar tissue and produces haemostasis during the initial stage of creation of the space in the retroperitoneum [22]. Though the conventional technique of retroperitoneoscopy has mostly been given up, it is still being used by some endosurgeons [8].

Indications

Retroperitoneoscopic nephrectomy is an ideal minimally invasive procedure for patients with small benign non-functioning symptomatic kidneys. It is also suitable for patients with end-stage renal disease requiring a pretransplant nephrectomy. It is not an ideal procedure for radical surgery in patients with renal malignancy as, due to limitation of space in the retroperitoneal area, there are more chances of the procedure being incomplete. Though it has also been used for a live donor nephrectomy, time alone will justify such an indication.

Patient selection

A thin patient with a hypoplastic kidney is an ideal patient for retroperitoneoscopic nephrectomy and should be selected when a surgeon is still relatively inexperienced. A patient with dense perinephric adhesions is best avoided as retroperitoneoscopic mobilization of such kidneys is time consuming and could even be dangerous.

Large cystic kidneys without much perinephric inflammatory adhesions can be easily removed after decompressing the kidney. Large solid kidneys are not at all suitable for retroperitoneoscopic removal as endoscopic manipulation is difficult due to the limited space available in the retroperitoneum.

The balloon dissection is difficult and unsatisfactory in the presence of fibrosis and, therefore, patients who have had retroperitoneal surgery done in the past should preferably be excluded. As the balloon performs an extensive retroperitoneal dissection, patients with bleeding disorders should also be excluded.

Preoperative preparation

Informed consent

The patients must be informed that though retroperitoneoscopic nephrectomy is slightly less invasive than its transperitoneal counterpart, it can also be associated with major vascular and visceral complications which could have serious consequences. They should also be told that the procedure may not be successful due to technical reasons and an open procedure might be required. A written consent must be obtained from all patients.

Preparation of the patient

All patients should have a routine medical checkup done to assess their fitness from a surgical and anaesthetic point of view. Antibiotic bowel preparation is not required, but a mechanical bowel preparation is advisable as a loaded colon might interfere in opening up the retroperitoneal space during the operative procedure. Prophylactic broad-spectrum antibiotics are administered 1 hour before the operation because of the potential risk of contamination associated with any laparoscopic procedure.

Preoperative procedures

Retroperitoneoscopic nephrectomy usually does not require any preoperative endoscopic procedure. Ureteral identification is easy after a good balloon dissection, but an exdwelling ureteral stent may be helpful in obese patients. A ureteral illuminator can also be used for the same purpose [23]. An indwelling urethral catheter is only inserted in patients requiring an additional total ureterectomy and a nasogastric tube is advisable in those having a right nephrectomy to keep the duodenum away.

Anaesthesia

All patients should have general endotrachial or regional anaesthesia. Local anaesthesia is not adequate for a retroperitoneal laparoscopic nephrectomy, as the extensive retroperitoneal dissection performed by the balloon can be quite painful and the muscle relaxation desirable during the operative procedure for adequate opening up of the retroperitoneal space may not be possible.

Surgical technique

The whole procedure of retroperitoneoscopic nephrectomy is described in the following 12 steps.

Positioning the patient (Fig. 6.1)
The patient is placed in a lateral kidney position and the kidney bridge is elevated to flatten out the lumbar region. A slight prone tilt of the patient is helpful in keeping the reflected peritoneum and the viscera out of the way, and in endoscopic surgical manipulation it helps by increasing the angle of the camera port in relation to the surgeon's working ports.

Location of the surgical team and the equipment (Fig. 6.2)
The surgeon sits facing the back of the patient while the nurse and second assistant stand on the other side. The latter moves towards the foot end of the patient as this makes it easier to handle the ports and to have a better view of the single monitor used by the surgeon. The first assistant is on the surgeon's side at the head end of the patient but moves to the foot end when the renal dissection is being performed. The monitor is on the other side near the head end at a height of about 1.5 m from the ground. The main instrument trolley is placed across the feet of the patient but another trolley with the frequently used instruments is kept on the right of the surgeon for convenience. The diathermy machine and the light source are kept on one side of the surgeon and the pneumoinsufflator on the other side.

Creation of the initial retroperitoneal space
After the patient has been prepped and draped, a standard subcostal 20 cm long kidney incision is marked see (see Fig. 6.1). A 2 cm skin incision is made along this line at its centre and is deepened by blunt dissection with an artery forceps down to the lumbodorsal fascia. The subrenal retroperitoneal space is entered by piercing the fascia with a sharp thrust of the artery forceps. The jaws of the forceps are opened and it is forced out to enlarge the gap in the fascia. The index or the little finger is introduced into the retroperitoneum and it is gently dissected to create a small space.

Figure 6.1
Position of the patient and location of the ports (right side). The dotted line is the standard subcostal kidney incision line. The incision for insertion of the balloon and the primary port (also called the balloon port) and the puncture sites for the two 10 mm ports (called the posterior and iliac ports) and a 5 mm port (called the anterior port) are shown.

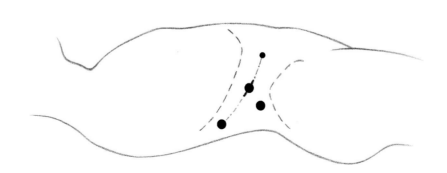

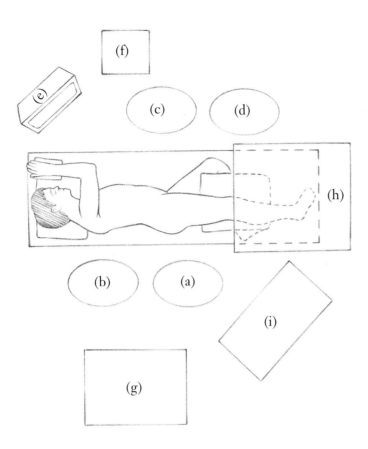

Subfascial placement of the balloon

The balloon is made by tying the palm or the finger portion of a surgical glove to a catheter or a commercially available balloon (Endo Exports, Bombay, India) can be used. Small deep retractors and fibreoptic light are used to expose the Gerota fascia in the depth of the retroperitoneal space already created. It is incised with scissors and the subfascial space is opened up with Hegar's dilators [5]. The balloon mounted on the feeding catheter is then manoeuvred into this subfascial perirenal space. If the balloon is bulky or if the tip of the feeding catheter is not extending up to its bottom, its placement can be facilitated by gently holding its tip with an artery forceps and stretching it.

In patients with small kidneys, obesity or chronic perinephric inflammation, it may be difficult to pick up the renal fascia and, therefore, in such cases the balloon is placed either deep to the fascia transversalis as for an upper ureterolithotomy or just outside the Gerota fascia. The anaesthetist can sometimes help the surgeon in picking up the Gerota fascia by providing a deep inspiratory pause.

Due to frequent problems of gas leakage around the balloon port, the author now places the balloon and the primary port percutaneously through a 10 mm incision just below the tip of the 12th rib as described in Chapter 7.

The balloon dissection

Using the pneumatic pump of a standard blood pressure apparatus, the balloon is inflated until it is bimanually palpable and almost touches the midline (about 30 pumpfuls). Fluid can also be used to inflate the balloon, especially by those who may have some objection to the use of air for fear of an air embolism following an explosive balloon rupture. We believe that the use of air to inflate the balloon is quite safe, provided it is a low pressure balloon. This is based on our clinical experience and the result of a recent study [24]. If the subfascial balloon pressure is more than 120 mmHg or if one is not sure about the balloon pressure, it is better to use fluid to inflate the balloon. This can be done with a 50 ml syringe using normal saline and it takes about 700–900 ml of the fluid for an adequate dissection in an adult.

Balloon pressures should be monitored during the early part of the learning curve to make sure that it is being inflated in a right plane. The subfascial balloon pressures in the balloons now used by us vary between 40 and 80 mmHg, depending upon the tissue resistance and the degree of distension. Normally, there is a gradual rise in the balloon pressure during inflation and sudden rise indicates that it is lying in an intermuscular or an interfascial plane and needs to be removed and reinserted. Apart from being economical and fast, the pneumatic pump also enables the operator to have a feel of the balloon pressure during inflation and with experience one can tell if it is being inflated in the right plane.

The balloon is left inflated for 5–7 minutes to allow for haemostasis to take place. Usually there is no bleeding around the balloon catheter during inflation indicating the atraumatic nature of the dissection, but if there is any bleeding it generally stops within 5 minutes. The balloon is thereafter deflated and removed.

Preliminary retroperitoneoscopy
A 10 mm cannula without a trocar is placed into the retroperitoneal space thus dissected and the opening is made airtight with a purse-string suture (Fig. 6.3) held with a haemostat [25]. A direct vision preliminary retroperitoneoscopy is performed with a 0° laparoscope and carbon dioxide insufflation at 10 mmHg pressure to assess the quality of the balloon dissection. If the surgeon is not happy with the quality or the extent of dissection, the balloon dissection can be repeated after placing it under vision or endoscopically deep to the fascia. Besides assessing the quality of balloon dissection, the area should also be carefully surveyed for any torn balloon pieces if there had been a balloon rupture.

In a thin patient with the balloon placed subfascially, one should be able to see a neatly dissected posterior surface of the kidney down to the renal capsule, most of the upper ureter, part of the inferior vena cava on the right side, and the psoas and quadratus lumborum muscles (Fig. 6.4). If the balloon is placed outside the fascia or if it slips out during inflation, or if the patient is quite obese, only the renal bulge and the muscles of the posterior abdominal wall will be identifiable.

Establishment of the ports
The laparoscope passed through the balloon port is attached to an endocamera after the preliminary retroperitoneoscopy has been performed. Two 10 mm ports, one at the posterior end of the marked kidney incision, the other just above the iliac crest and a third 5 mm port at the anterior end of the marked incision, are established under vision as accessory ports (see Fig 6.1). While placing the anterior port, the surgeon sometimes may not be sure of a safe entry due to the overlying fat camouflaging a fold of peritoneum or colon. In such cases, we prefer the use of a digital guidance technique [22]. The left index finger is placed inside the retroperitoneal space through the 20 mm incision and is used to strip the

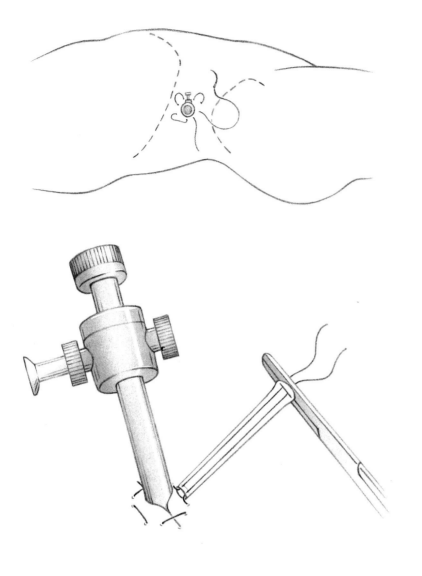

Figure 6.3
Placement of a purse-string suture. The two ends of the proline suture, passed through a tube made out of a sheath of a disposable hypodermic needle, are kept in position with an artery forceps to make the incision airtight around the primary port.

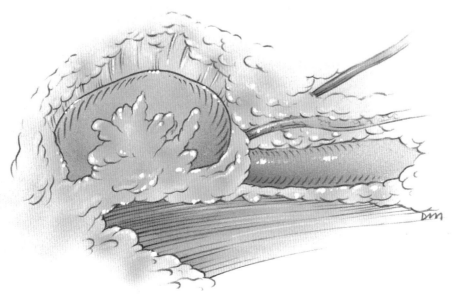

Figure 6.4
View of the right retroperitoneum after a good balloon dissection. The posterior surface of the kidney, the upper ureter, the internal spermatic vein, part of the inferior vena cava, the psoas muscle, the renal pelvis covered with fat, the reflected posterior peritoneum and the adrenal with overlying fat can be seen.

abdominal wall of the suspected peritoneum or colon. The trocar is placed directly at the tip of the index finger while it is lifting the abdominal wall and the trocar is then guided safely into the retroperitoneal space by the finger (Fig. 6.5). The two posterior ports can also be similarly established. To prevent injury to the tip of the finger, one can use a finger guard, but we prefer the use of slightly blunt trocars.

For retroperitoneal punctures, there is no need to have very sharp trocars as one does not have to go through the peritoneum or tough fascial layers. The blunt trocars also reduce the risk of accidental visceral or vascular damage. They should not be longer than 18 cm in view of the small space available in the retroperitoneum. This also provides an easy palmar grip and the use of the index finger as a safety stopper.

Dissection and division of the ureter
The upper ureter is easily identified due to its peristaltic activity following a subfascial balloon dissection. It is grabbed with a 5 mm endo-Babcock through the iliac port and is dissected up to the ureteropelvic junction using a 5 mm spatula dissector through the posterior port (Fig 6.6). This dissection is through an avascular plane and usually there is no significant bleeding. However, if there are any doubtful vascular strands, they should be electrocoagulated. The ureter is clip ligated through the posterior port at the desired level and is divided between the clips.

If the ureter is not visible, it is endoscopically explored by blunt dissection over the psoas muscle with simultaneous lifting up of the posterior peritoneum with a retractor. In case of any difficulty, it should be searched for in the area between the renal sinus and the lower pole of the kidney. If any problem in

Figure 6.5
Placement of accessory ports by the digital guidance technique. The left index finger, after stripping the peritoneum away, raises a fold of the anterior abdominal wall and guides the trocar safely into the retroperitoneal space.

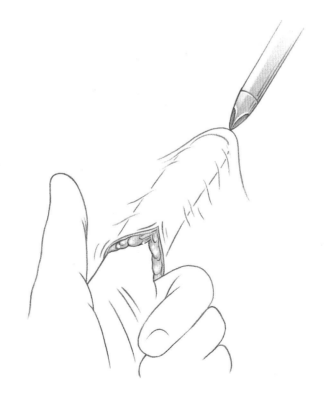

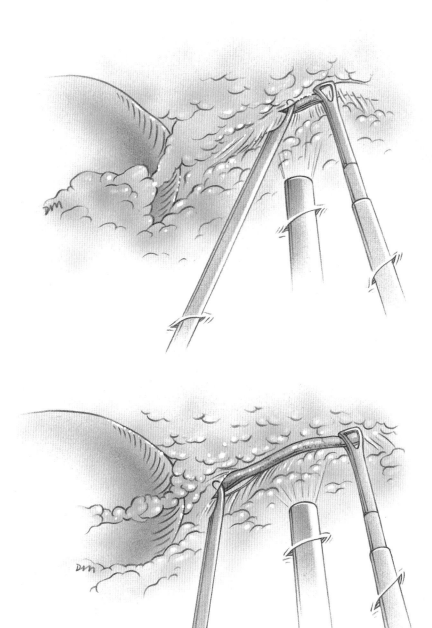

Figure 6.6
Dissection of the upper right ureter. It is grabbed with a 5 mm Babcock through the iliac port and is stripped of its sheath with a 5 mm spatula dissector through the posterior port. The camera is at the balloon port. The kidney is also seen.

ureteral identity is anticipated due to obesity, retroperitoneal inflammatory disease or ureteral atresia, the ureter should be stented preoperatively. If the ureter still cannot be identified or if the kidney is lying low, it is better to leave the ureter untouched until the end of the procedure.

Dissection of the kidney

If the posterior surface of the kidney has been dissected by the balloon, there is no definite order in which it should be dissected further. However, irrespective of whether it has been dissected by the balloon or not, we usually dissect the posterior surface, the lower pole, the upper pole, the anterior surface and the pedicle in that order.

Any residual perinephric fat on the posterior surface of the kidney is stripped away, but if the kidney has not been dissected by the balloon, the Gerota fascia is divided using an endoshear through the right posterior port (i.e. the iliac port for a right nephrectomy and the posterior port for a left nephrectomy) and an endoforceps through the left posterior port (Fig. 6.7). The posterior surface of the kidney is then completely dissected down to the renal capsule using a combination of sharp and blunt dissection. A 10 mm blunt spatula dissector (Kalelkar Surgicals, Bombay, India) is a multipurpose instrument for atraumatic blunt dissection, retraction and ligation of the renal pedicle and we have found it to be quite useful in dissecting kidneys with little perinephric inflammation (Fig 6.8). For adherent kidneys, sharp dissection is mostly required and it is best done with an endoshear with or without the use of cautery. For blunt dissection, a pneumodissector has also been used successfully [26], but the author does not have any personal experience.

The lower pole of the kidney is then completely dissected starting with the lower border, followed by the lateral border, the medial border and the anterior surface, in that order. The internal spermatic vein, if encountered, should be clip ligated and any doubtful vascular strands electrocoagulated. For dissection of the anterior surface, while the first assistant retracts the posterior peritoneum away through the anterior port, the surgeon pulls the kidney posteriorly with the 10 mm blunt spatula to provide a better exposure of the area (Fig 6.9). The upper pole is then dissected in a similar way by pulling it down with the blunt spatula, taking care not to damage the suprarenal gland. The duodenum and the inferior vena cava present at various phases of the medial dissection on the right side and should be carefully preserved.

The anterior surface of the remaining kidney is dissected at the end, in a way similar to the one described for the lower pole. Apart from the duodenum and the inferior vena cava on the right side, care should also be taken not to damage the posterior peritoneum, the colon, the pancreas and the renal vein or its tributaries.

Figure 6.7
Exposure of the kidney if it has not been dissected by the balloon. The perinephric fat is seen as Gerota's fascia and is divided with an endoshear through the iliac port, an endoforceps through the posterior port and the camera through the balloon port. The psoas is the only clearly identifiable landmark.

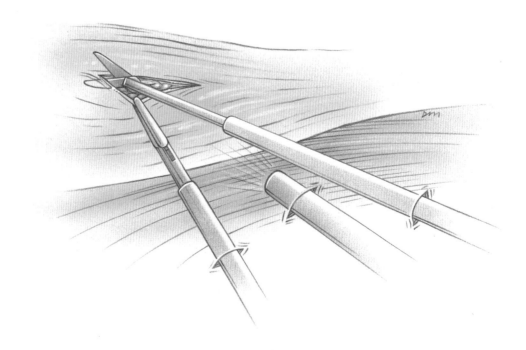

(a)

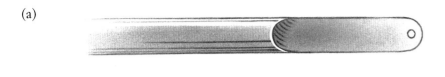

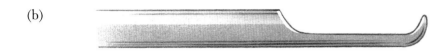

(b)

Figure 6.8
The multipurpose dissector–retractor–ligature carrier: (a) front view, and (b) side view.

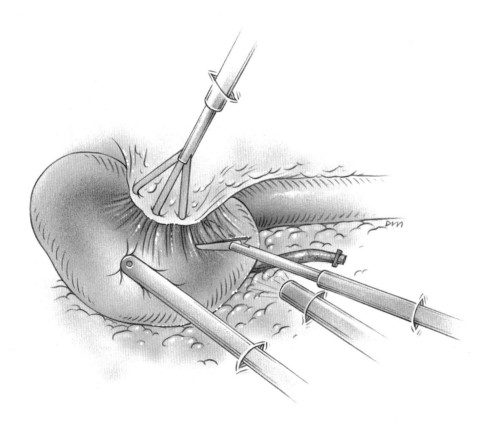

Figure 6.9
Dissection of the anterior surface of the kidney. The posterior peritoneum and the duodenum are retracted through the anterior port, the kidney is pushed down with the 10 mm multipurpose instrument, and the areolar adhesions divided with an endoshear through the iliac port. The inferior vena cava and the divided ureter are also seen.

Sometimes it may be difficult to identify retroperitoneoscopically a small atrophic, hypoplastic or a multicystic kidney without any renal parenchyma. In such patients, rather than groping in the dark and risking visceral or peritoneal damage, it is much safer to follow the ureter up to the kidney. The kidney, being small, can be easily handled in these patients by holding the ureteral stump and there is hardly any point in using a retractor for the kidney.

Dissection and division of the pedicle
The first assistant lifts the kidney up by pulling the ureteral stump if the kidney is small, and by using a retractor through the anterior port if it is large. For a better

view of the pedicle, the laparoscope can be shifted to the iliac port and the balloon port used by the surgeon for endoscopic dissection. Being posterior, the renal artery is dissected first and it can be easily identified in the cephalic part of the pedicle due to its pulsations. This dissection should be done very carefully using an endoshear and an endodissector, with judicious use of electocautery. The renal artery can be more easily dissected if the assistant makes it taut by giving extra lift to the kidney. A blunt 7 mm hook helps in atraumatic stripping of the artery and it can also be used for steadying the artery for clip ligation (Fig. 6.10). Three clips are applied to the artery proximally and one clip is applied near the

Figure 6.10
(a) Dissection of the pedicle. The kidney is retracted up through the anterior port, the endoforceps lifts the areolar tissue over the renal pedicle through the posterior port , and the endoshear carefully divides it through the iliac port. The divided ureter can also be seen with the camera through the balloon port. (b) Same as figure (a) except that a 7 mm blunt hook through the iliac port pulls the renal artery for clip ligating it through the posterior port.

(a)

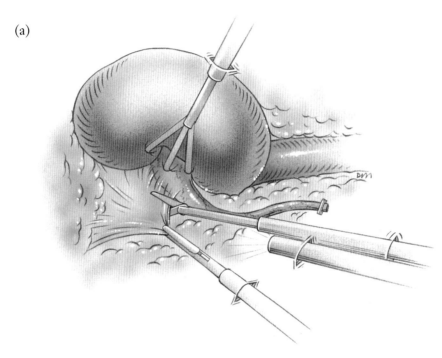

(b)

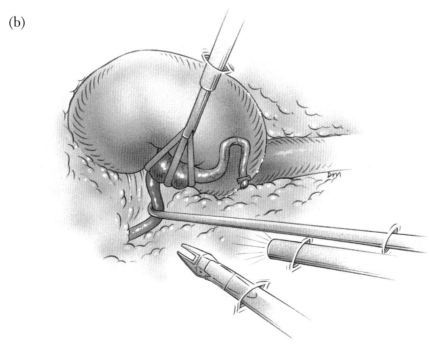

kidney and the artery is then divided between the clips. Rarely, the artery is large for the clips and under such circumstances it can either be ligated endoscopically or an endo-GIA can be used. We prefer the use of the multipurpose instrument for taking the ligature around the pedicle and for tying the knots [3]. Following this, the renal vein or veins are likewise dissected, clip ligated and divided.

It is easy to damage a lumbar vein during dissection of the pedicle and the bleeding can sometimes be frightening. Luckily, the bleeding can be controlled in most cases by using a rapid sequence clip applicator or by packing through the balloon port incision.

Extraction of the kidney

To make sure that the kidney has been made totally free, it is grabbed with a 10 mm endo-Babcock, rotated two to three times and then pushed down in the iliac fossa. Small benign non-infected kidneys are then removed through the balloon port incision in the following way. The ureter is grabbed with an endo-Babcock through the anterior port. The balloon is removed and the purse-string suture is pulled out. The skin incision is extended by 1–2 cm and the opening is enlarged by stretching the muscles with small right-angled retractors. The endo-Babcock holding the ureter is pushed through the enlarged incision using the digital guidance technique. The ureter is pulled out and the endo-Babcock is removed. The lower pole of the kidney is held with a sponge-holding forceps and it is pulled out using to and fro motions as the assistant stretches the opening with a pair of small retractors. If the kidney is lost by accidental tearing off of the ureter, it can be grabbed endoscopically with a sponge-holding forceps passed directly through the enlarged incision, after making it partially leakproof by packing it with a sponge.

If the kidney is large, infected or neoplastic, it is placed in a lapsac (Cook Urological, Spencer, Indiana, USA) and is pulled out after morcellation with a 10 mm cup forceps or a sponge-holding forceps, but without extending the incision. Mechanical or electrical morcellators are really not necessary for the type of kidneys removed retroperitoneoscopically.

Closure of the ports

The retroperitoneal space is irrigated with normal saline through the balloon port incision to flush out loose fibrofatty tissue and blood clots. It is then gently mopped with small gauze pieces through the same incision to check for any bleeding and to remove residual tissue debris. Any active bleeding is dealt with endoscopically, after making the incision airtight with a sponge. A glove drain is passed through the posterior port at the end of the procedure. The 5 mm incision is closed with a single cutaneous stitch, while the 10 mm ones are closed in two layers using absorbable suture material.

Postoperative care

The patients are ambulatory and allowed oral feeds the same evening. The urethral catheter and the nasogastric tube, if any, are removed after the operative procedure. Patients are usually discharged from the hospital the day after removing the glove drain. Broad-spectrum antibiotics are given routinely for 5 days postoperatively. Oral analgesics are usually required for 2–4 days and patients can resume non-strenuous activity within 2 weeks.

Clinical experience

Though a large number of nephrectomies have been performed retroperitoneoscopically, only 43 have so far been reported [27–33]. Retroperitoneoscopic nephrectomies were performed by us in 15 patients during the last 3 years. One patient had a multicystic kidney, three had hypoplastic kidneys with recurrent infection (one with prune-belly syndrome), six had chronic calculus disease, two had primary ureteropelvic junction obstruction, two had end-stage renal disease with chronic pyelonephritis and one was a live kidney donor with a normal kidney. Four patients had large hydronephrotic kidneys (12–17 cm long) and 10 had small kidneys (6–8 cm long). The age ranged between 10 and 50 years and the mean age was 27 years. There were three children under the age of 15 years old and all the patients were of average Indian build.

There were two failures due to dense perinephric adhesions in patients with large kidneys: these were converted into mini open procedures by joining two of the three incisions placed along the marked kidney incision. The kidney was almost completely mobilized retroperitoneoscopically in the live donor without any ischaemic damage, but the division of the ureter and the renal pedicle and the removal of the kidney was done through a 15 cm incision.

In 12 patients, nephrectomy was performed successfully using the retroperitoneoscopic technique, but one conversion to the transperitoneal technique was required due to the kidney being large. All kidneys were removed after enlarging the balloon port incision by one or two centimetres. The average operative time was about 2 hours. Eight patients were discharged the next day, and two were kept longer due to end-stage renal disease and two due to socioeconomical reasons. Oral analgesics were used by all for up to 4 days.

There were only some minor complications in this series. A large hydronephrotic kidney was accidentally punctured with the artery forceps in a patient during the creation of the initial retroperitoneal space but was of no consequence. There was bleeding during dissection of the pedicle from a torn lumbar vein, and the procedure had to be converted into an open one. Two patients had surgical emphysema extending to the face, which settled down within a few hours.

The experience of other workers has more or less been identical. Chiu et al. had two open conversions and no major complications in their 14 patients who had retroperitoneal laparoscopic nephrectomies [27] using the balloon technique. Similarly, in Gill and colleagues' series of 12 nephrectomies (one partial and one with ureterectomy) performed with the same technique, no major complications were reported [28]. Munch et al. even performed bilateral nephrectomy in a patient in a similar way without any morbidity [29]. Wolf et al. reported greater absorption of carbon dioxide in patients undergoing retroperitoneal laparoscopic renal surgery compared to transperitoneal surgery [34], while Chiu et al., in an experimental study, found significant systemic and renal haemodynamic changes during retroperitoneal pneumoinsufflation, though it was of a lesser degree compared to the transperitoneal procedure [35].

Conclusion

Retroperitoneal endoscopic nephrectomy using the balloon technique of retroperitoneoscopy is safe, simple and fairly reliable. Due to the limited space available in the retroperitoneum it is not suitable for larger kidneys, which are better removed transperitoneally. Being used to the direct posterior extraperitoneal approach, which does not involve mobilization of the colon, most surgeons feel more comfortable with the retroperitoneoscopic approach. It also has the advantage of exposing and ligating the renal artery before the renal vein is encountered which may not be possible with the transperitoneal approach.

The author's balloon technique of retroperitoneoscopy does not involve blind trocar and Veress needle punctures and is therefore theoretically safer than other contemporary retroperitoneal endoscopic techniques. The balloon provides a good start for the endoscopic surgeon by performing a neat dissection of the kidney and the ureter if placed deep to the renal fascia.

References

1   Clayman RV, Kavoussi LR, Soper NJ *et al*. Laparoscopic nephrectomy: initial case report. *J Urol* 1991; **146**: 278–81.
2   Clayman RV, Kavoussi LR, Soper NJ *et al*. Laparoscopic nephrectomy: review of the initial 10 cases. *J Endourol* 1992; **6**: 127–31.
3   Gaur DD, Agarwal DK, Purohit KC. Retroperitoneal laparoscopic nephrectomy: initial case report. *J Urol* 1993; **149**: 103–5.
4   Gaur DD. Laparoscopic operative retroperitoneoscopy: use of a new device. *J Urol* 1992; **148**: 1137–9.
5   Gaur DD. The use of Hegar's dilator in laparoscopy. *J Min Inv Therapy* 1993; **2**: 333–4.
6   Gaur DD, Agarwal DK, Purohit KC, Darshane AS. Retroperitoneal laparoscopic pyelolithotomy. *J Urol* 1994; **154**: 927–9.
7   Gaur DD, Agarwal DK, Purohit KC, Darshane AS, Shah BC. Retroperitoneal laparoscopic ureterolithotomy for multiple upper mid ureteral calculi. *J Urol* 1994; **151**: 1001–2.
8   Mandressi A, Buizza C, Zaroli A *et al*. Laparoscopic nephrectomies and adrenalectomies by posterior retro-extra-peritoneal approach (abstract WX-4). *J Endourol* 1993; **7**(Suppl.): S174.
9   Rassweiler JJ, Henkel TO, Potempa DM, Becker P, Alken P. Laparoscopic retroperitoneal nephrectomy (abstract V-122). *J Endourol* 1993; **7**(Suppl.): S230.
10   Chandhoke PS, Galansky S, Koyle M, Kaula NF. Pediatric retroperitoneal nephrectomy (abstract PXII-12). *J Endourol* 1993; **7**(Suppl.): S138.
11   Clayman RV, McDougall EM, Kerbal K, Anderson K, Kavoussi LR. Laparoscopic nephrectomy: transperitoneal vs retroperitoneal (abstract PXII-15). *J Endourol* 1993; **7**(Suppl.): S139.
12   Munch LC, Gill IS. Laparoscopic retroperitoneal partial nephrectomy for stone disease (abstract V-116). *J Endourol* 1993; **7**(Suppl.): S228.
13   Gaur DD, Agarwal DK, Purohit KC, Darshane AS, Saxena VK. Retroperitoneal laparoscopic decortication of renal cyst (abstract V-112). *J Endourol* 1993; **7**(Suppl.): S227.
14   Wong HY, Griffith DP. Renal cyst marsupialization via retroperitoneoscopy (abstract V-114). *J Endourol* 1993; **7**(Suppl.): S228.
15   Gaur DD, Agarwal DK, Purohit KC. Retroperitoneal laparoscopic renoscopy and renal biopsy (abstract PXII-4). *J Endourol* 1993; **7**(Suppl.): S136.
16   Harewood LM, Webb DR, Pope A. Retroperitoneal laparoscopic ureterolithotomy utilizing balloon dilatation of the retroperitoneum (abstract V-160). *J Endourol* 1993; **7**(Suppl.): S239.
17   Munch LC, Delworth MG, Gill IS. Retroperitoneal laparoscopic ureterolithotomy (abstract PXII-5). *J Endourol* 1993; **7**(Suppl.): S137.
18   Gaur DD, Agarwal DK, Purohit KC *et al*. Laparoscopic ureterolithotomy: our experience in 17 patients. *Bombay Hosp J* 1993; **35**: 65–8.
19   Gaur DD, Agarwal DK, Purohit KC, Darshane AS. Retroperitoneal laparoscopic pyelolithotomy and pyeloplasty (abstract V-151). *J Endourol* 1993; **7**(Suppl.): S237.
20   Gaur DD, Saxena VK, Nair KR, Agarwal DK, Pain CR. Retroperitoneal laparoscopic adrenalectomy (abstract PXII-2). *J Endourol* 1993; **7**(Suppl.): S136.
21   Williams PL, Warwick R. Myology. In: Williams PL, Warwick R, eds. *Gray's Anatomy*, 36th edn. Edinburgh: Churchill Livingstone, 1980: 506–93.

22 Gaur DD. Retroperitoneoscopy: the balloon technique. *Ann R Coll Surg Engl* 1994; **76**: 259–63.
23 Kirkali Z, Esen AA, Celebi I. An easy way of ureteral identification: ureteral illuminator (abstract VI-42). *J Endourol* 1994; **8**(Suppl.): S55.
24 Gaur DD, Agarwal DK, Kulkarni SB, Purohit KC, Shah HK. Retroperitoneoscopy: the dynamics of balloon dissection. Presented to the BAUS annual meeting, Birmingham, UK, July 1994.
25 Gaur DD. Retroperitoneal laparoscopy: some technical modifications. *Br J Urol* (in press).
26 Clayman RV, Fadden PT, McDougall EM *et al*. Pneumodissection: a new method of laparoscopic tissue dissection (abstract PXII-12). *J Endoural* 1993; **7**(Suppl): S197.
27 Chiu AW, Chou C, Wang B *et al*. Retroperitoneoscopic nephrectomy for the treatment of nonfunctioning kidneys (abstract P1-65). *J Endourol* 1994; **7**(Suppl.): S79.
28 Gill IS, Das S, Munch LC. Retroperitoneoscopy: a viable alternative (abstract P4-135). *J Endourol* 1994; **7**(Suppl.): S91.
29 Munch LC, Gill IS, Miller SG, Lucas BA. Bilateral retroperitoneal laparoscopic native nephrectomy following renal transplantation (abstract P1-72). *J Endourol* 1994; **7**(Suppl.): S81.
30 Koyle M, Chandhoke P, Galansky S. Pediatric retroperitoneal laparoscopic nephrectomy (abstract P5-148). *J Endourol* 1994; **7**(Suppl.): S94.
31 Schulman CC, Jansen T, Rassweiler J. Retroperitoneal laparoscopic nephrectomy in children. Presented to the SIU annual meeting, Sydney, Australia, September 1994.
32 Rassweiler J, Henkel TO, Stock *et al*. Retroperitoneoscopy for ablative and reconstructive procedures. Presented to the SIU annual meeting, Sydney, Australia, September 1994.
33 Gaur DD. Retroperitoneal surgery of the kidney, ureter and adrenal. *Endosc Surg* 1995; **3**: 3–8.
34 Wolf IS, Monk TG, McDougall EM, Clayman RV. The extraperitoneal approach and subcutaneous emphysema are associated with greater absorption of CO_2 during laparoscopic surgery (abstract P5-145). *J Endourol* 1994; **7**(Suppl.) S93.
35 Chiu AW, Chang LS, Birkett DH, Babayan RK. Effects of pneumoperitoneum and pneumoretroperitoneum on systemic and renal hemodynamics (abstract O3-37). *J Endourol* 1994; **7**(Suppl.): S54.

Chapter 7

Retroperitoneoscopy and ureteric surgery

D.D. Gaur

Introduction

Though Wickham performed a retroperitoneal laparoscopic ureterolithotomy as early as 1979 [1], no further progress could be made in this direction, due to mostly unsuccessful results of past retroperitoneoscopies, until the author described his balloon technique of retroperitoneoscopy in 1992 [2]. This was because of failure to realize that the retroperitoneum, being abundant in tough areolar and fibrofatty tissue, would not yield to Veress needle insufflation [3].

Due to the poor results of retroperitoneoscopy in the past, Clayman *et al.* performed a percutaneous ureterolithotomy after dilating a percutaneously established track under fluoroscopic control [4] and Meretyk *et al.* reported the removal of a foreign body lodged near the ureter using a similar technique [5]. It was only after realizing the potentials of the balloon technique of retroperitoneoscopy, that attention was once again drawn towards the retroperitoneal endoscopic approach to the ureter.

Indications

Retroperitoneoscopy provides a good exposure of the whole ureter, especially in its upper and mid part and therefore can be used for any type of ureteral surgery. The main indication for retroperitoneoscopic ureteric surgery is ureterolithotomy, but it can also be used for ureterostomy, ureterolysis, ureteral reimplantation and the management of ureteral stricture, primary ureteropelvic junction obstruction or retrocaval ureter.

Ureterostomy can be performed as a temporary procedure for grossly dilated, poorly draining ureters or as a permanent procedure for urinary incontinence due to advanced pelvic malignancy. Ureterolysis is a simple retroperitoneoscopic procedure for localized periureteral fibrosis, but for advanced retroperitoneal fibrosis the procedure may be difficult or even impossible. Ureteral reimplantation could be a difficult procedure retroperitoneoscopically due to the truncated retroperitoneal space in the pelvis and is better performed transperitoneally [6].

Resection of a ureteral stricture or Davis' intubated ureterotomy can be performed by this approach, but the surgeon has to have a lot of experience in endoscopic suturing techniques. The newer endoscopic glueing techniques appear to have a great potential in making these procedures simpler and faster [7]. Ureteropelvic junction obstructions and retrocaval ureters can also be managed similarly [8,9].

Retroperitoneal laparoscopic ureterolithotomy is indicated in the following situations:

1 When extracorporeal shockwave lithotripsy (ESWL) and endourological facilities are not available.
2 When the calculi are not amenable to ESWL or endourological procedures due to their size, hardness and impaction.
3 When the calculus is associated with a stricture of the ureter.

In many developing countries, though endourological and ESWL facilities may not be available, laparoscopic equipment is easily accessible due to the government policy of encouraging the family planning programme. Retroperitoneal laparoscopic ureterolithotomy is the most suitable minimally invasive therapeutic procedure, under such circumstances, as an alternative to an open surgical procedure.

A small percentage of ureteral calculi are not amenable to ESWL or an endourological procedure as they are large, hard and chronically impacted. Retroperitoneal laparoscopic ureterolithotomy can be easily utilized as a salvage procedure in these patients. It can also be recommended as a primary procedure in a select group of patients, where one anticipates multiple sittings of ESWL and endourological procedures or where exposure to radiation is not advisable. While deciding on the modality of treatment to be used for a particular patient, it must be borne in mind that the more difficult a stone is to treat by ESWL and endourology, the easier it is to treat by retroperitoneal laparoscopic ureterolithotomy.

A calculus associated with a ureteral stricture can be treated by endourological procedures, but retroperitoneal laparoscopy provides an easy access for performing a simultaneous Davis' intubated ureterotomy or even resection of the stricture and ureteroureterostomy.

Patient selection

A thin patient with a large impacted calculus in the upper ureter is an ideal case for the beginner surgeon. With more experience in the field of retroperitoneoscopy, patients with obesity and lower ureteral impaction can also be considered for this procedure.

As mentioned in Chapter 6, patients who have had retroperitoneal surgery performed previously and those with bleeding disorders should preferably be excluded.

Preoperative preparation

Informed consent

This should be obtained from all patients and they should be told about the possibility of complications and the risk involved.

Preparation of the patient

This is similar to the one performed for the nephrectomy patients (see Chapter 6), but as the lithotomy patients are prone to urinary tract infection and obstructive uropathy, a urine culture should be done routinely and an appropriate antibiotic given as per the sensitivity report. If it is associated with an acute obstruction, percutaneous nephrostomy drainage should be performed. If the surgeon is relatively inexperienced, it is recommended that a plain X-ray of the abdomen is taken with a coin strapped to the umblicus as this provides a bearing for locating the calculus endoscopically.

Preoperative procedures

Retroperitoneoscopic ureterolithotomy very rarely requires a preoperative endoscopic procedure as there is little problem in ureteral identification, except in obese patients where an exdwelling ureteral stent may be helpful. Preoperative placement of a double-J stent, though helpful in identifying the ureter during the endoscopic procedure, is usually not possible in these patients as the calculi are mostly impacted. A double-J stent assembly can be passed up to the calculus in patients with upper ureteral calculi and advanced further intraoperatively after the calculus has been removed, if one intends keeping it postoperatively. An indwelling urethral catheter is only necessary for procedures on the pelvic ureter and a nasogastric tube is not required.

Anaesthesia

A general or regional anaesthesia with adequate muscle relaxation is desirable.

Surgical technique

There are two types of retroperitoneoscopic approach to the ureter. The lumbar approach is used for calculi in the upper and mid-ureter, and the iliac one for those in the lower and lower mid-ureter.

Lumbar approach

Positioning the patient
The patient is placed in a lateral position and the kidney bridge is elevated to open out the lumbar region. In patients with mid-ureteral calculi a slight supine tilt of the pelvis keeps it out of the way during endoscopic surgical manipulation.

Location of the surgical team and the equipment
For an upper ureterolithotomy the placement of the equipment and the positioning of the surgical team is identical to the one for a retroperitoneoscopic nephrectomy (see Chapter 6). For a mid-ureterolithotomy, there is an exchange in the positions of the surgeon with the first assistant and monitor with the second assistant (Fig. 7.1). The nurse moves to the other side of the patient to keep clear of the monitor.

Figure 7.1
Location of the surgical team and the equipment for a right mid ureterolithotomy: (a) surgeon, (b) first assistant, (c) second assistant, (d) nurse, (e) monitor, (f) pneumoinsufflator, (g) diathermy machine, (h) main instrument trolley, and (i) frequently used instrument trolley.

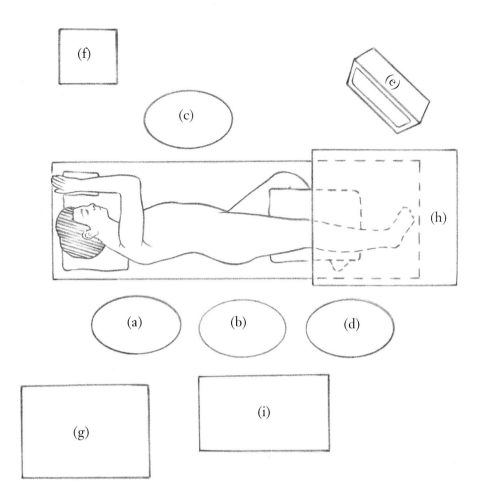

Creation of the initial retroperitoneal space
This is absolutely identical to the one described for patients undergoing retroperitoneoscopic nephrectomy (see Chapter 6). We now use a percutaneous technique for the insertion of the balloon and the primary port in all our patients (Fig. 7.2).

Retroperitoneal placement of the balloon
The balloon used is similar to the one used for a nephrectomy patient. Using small deep retractors and a fibreoptic light, the fascia transversalis is picked up with artery forceps and is brought out to the skin level with or without further dissection. It is incised with scissors (Fig. 7.3) and the retroperitoneal space deep to the fascia transversalis is opened up with Hegar's dilators [10]. The balloon is then placed into this space.

The subfascial placement of the balloon is quite easy in thin patients, but may be difficult or even impossible in obese patients or in those with chronic retroperitoneal inflammatory disease. Under such circumstances the balloon is placed outside the fascia in the retroperitoneal space created initially by digital dissection.

(a)

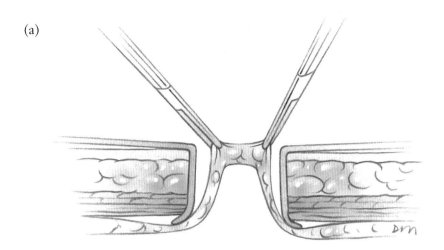

Figure 7.2
*Creation of initial
retroperitoneal space (a) The
fascia transversalis has been
picked up with haemostats,
after retracting with small
deep retractors. A fold of
parietal peritoneum can also
be pulled up with the fascia
in thin patients. (b) The
fascia is cut with scissors and
a Hegar's dilator is used to
open up the space between the
fascia and the peritoneum.*

(b)

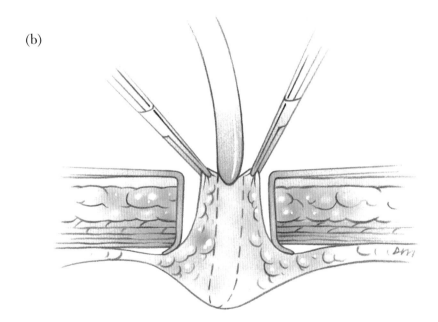

The balloon dissection
The balloon should be manipulated in a slightly cephaled direction for an upper
ureteral calculus and in a caudal direction for a mid-ureteral calculus. It is then
gradually inflated with air or fluid as described in Chapter 6, until the balloon
bulge in the lumbar region touches the midline for an upper ureteric calculus or
migrates to the iliac region for a mid-ureteric calculus. This usually requires
about 700 ml of fluid for an upper ureteric calculus and 900 ml for a mid-ureteric
calculus. If undue force is being required to inflate the balloon, it could be either
due to a kink in the feeding catheter or placement of the balloon in a wrong
plane. The former can be ascertained by a poor retrograde flow from the balloon
and can be corrected by slightly pulling out the catheter. If there is no kink in the
catheter, the balloon has to be in a wrong plane and it should be taken out and

Figure 7.3

The percutaneous technique of inserting the balloon and the primary port. (a) A blunt artery forceps is pushed down into the subrenal retroperitoneal space through a 10 mm incision below the tip of the 12th rib. (b) The track is dilated with a 10 mm blunt obturator and the retroperitoneal space is blindly dissected by a to and fro movement of the obturator over the psoas muscle. (c) Using the same blunt obturator, a 10 mm cannula is introduced into the retroperitoneal space and direct visual (or by using an endocamera) dissection of the retroperitoneum is performed to create a space under the fascia transversalis or the Gerota fascia using the tip of the telescope as a dissector. (d) The cannula is positioned in the space to be dissected, the telescope is removed and the balloon mounted on a catheter is introduced into the retroperitoneum through the 10 mm cannula. The cannula is removed before the balloon is inflated.

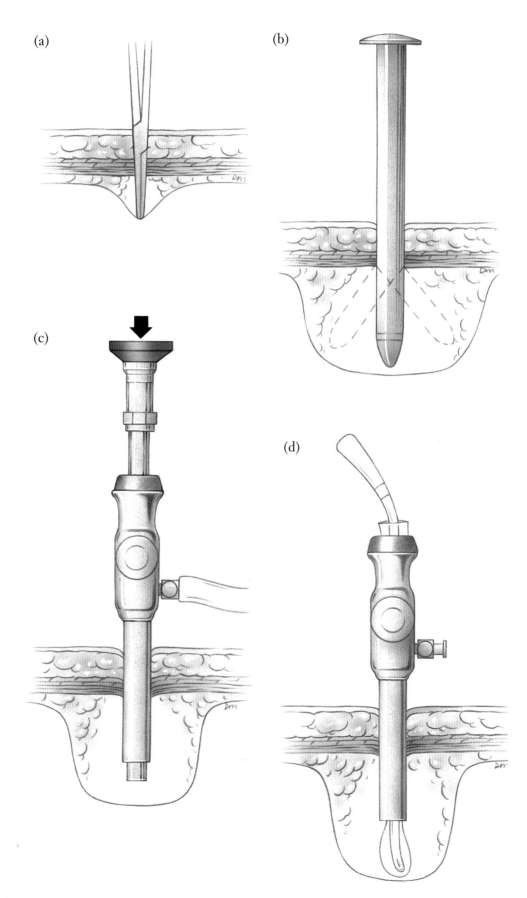

(a)

(b)

(c)

(d)

reinserted. After the balloon has been fully inflated, it should be left in place for 5–7 minutes and then deflated and removed to allow for haemostasis to take place.

Preliminary retroperitoneoscopy
This is performed to assess the quality of the retroperitoneal dissection and to have some bearings before the endoscopic dissection is started. During a repeat balloon dissection, if one feels that the balloon is not migrating towards the area of interest during inflation, it can be manipulated abdominally by applying counterpressure in the area of unwanted migration. If this also does not help, a digital dissection or an endoscopic dissection using the tip of the telescope is performed towards the area of interest, before reinserting the balloon for a repeat dissection.

After a good balloon dissection, one should be able to see a neatly dissected lower pole of the kidney, the whole of the upper ureter, the internal spermatic vein approaching the ureter at an acute angle, the inferior vena cava, the common iliac artery and the psoas and quadratus lumborum muscles. With the balloon placed outside the fascia, one may not be able to identify anything except the muscles of the posterior abdominal wall as they remain hidden by the overlying fascia, which often cannot be disrupted by the balloon. In such circumstances the ureter can be identified either by the stone bulge or by the indwelling stent. Otherwise, one has to search for it using blunt dissection endoscopically. To prevent the balloon slipping out during inflation, the artery forceps holding the edges of the fascia transversalis are crossed over the balloon and left hanging, on each side of the feeding catheter (Fig. 7.4),

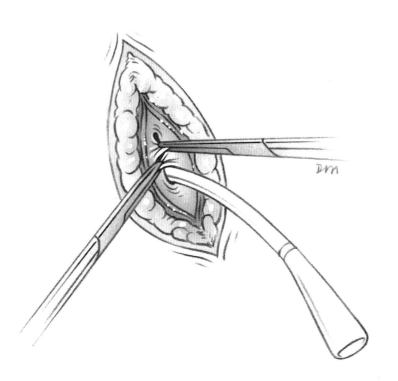

Figure 7.4
The artery forceps holding the edges of the fascia transversalis are crossed over and allowed to hang on each side of the feeding catheter to prevent the balloon slipping out.

Establishment of the ports

Two 10 mm and one 5 mm ports are established at the ends of the kidney incision line and just above the iliac crest, as described in Chapter 6.

Dissection of the ureter

If the ureter has already been dissected and the calculus is in its upper part, the ureter is grabbed above or below the stone bulge with an endo-Babcock through the iliac port which is steadied by the assistant. The first assistant manages the camera and helps in changing the instruments, while the second assistant uses the anterior port to retract the posterior peritoneum. The surgeon uses the iliac and the posterior ports to further dissect the stone-bearing ureter, mostly by blunt dissection. Electrocoagulation is rarely required as there is hardly any bleeding. For procedures on the mid-ureter, a 30° laparoscope, if available, makes the dissection easier.

If the ureter cannot be identified following the balloon dissection, it is explored by a combination of blunt and sharp dissection starting above or below the visible or expected stone bulge. If the stone is lower down, sometimes it may be difficult to locate the ureter endoscopically, but a dilated ureter usually poses no problem of identification. The blunt dissection of the ureter should be performed from above downwards to prevent the stone from getting dislodged and migrating to the pelvicalyceal system.

Suction and irrigation is usually not required during ureteral dissection. If it is needed it is often not effective due to frequent clogging by free floating fat and areolar tissue. We have found the sump suction used for open abdominal operations to be quite useful [11]. It easily goes through a 10 mm port and does a good job inspite of it being a blind procedure (Fig. 7.5).

Removal of the calculus

The dilated ureter is grabbed about 1 cm proximal to the stone with the endo-Babcock positioned through the iliac port. The endo-Babcock is pressed down against the psoas muscle so that the stone-bearing part is lying obliquely (Fig. 7.6). If this is not possible in a grossly dilated ureter, it is grabbed distal to the calculis. Using a retractable endoknife (Cook Urological, Spencer, Indiana, USA) through the posterior port, the ureter is incised over 5 mm of proximal ureter and 75% of the calculus. The stone is mobilized by freeing it of the ureteral adhesions with a 5 mm spatula dissector and it is then levered out of the ureter. If not very large, it is engulfed by a 10 mm cup forceps and is removed through the posterior port (Fig. 7.7). If large, it is pushed out through the balloon port after removing the cannula and loosening the purse-string suture or by slightly enlarging one of the ports.

The calculus in the mid-ureter is removed in a similar way, except that the endo-Babcock passed through the iliac port holds the ureter distal to the calculus to prevent crossing of the swords [12].

Ureteral flushing

The ureteral incision is flushed with normal saline using a curved tip 5 mm ureteral flushing cannula to remove residual stone pieces. In patients with upper ureteral calculi, the pelvicalyceal system can also be flushed by introducing a 3–4 cm length of a 12F catheter attached to the tip of the flushing cannula (Fig. 7.8). The same catheter can also be used to test the patency of the distal ureter.

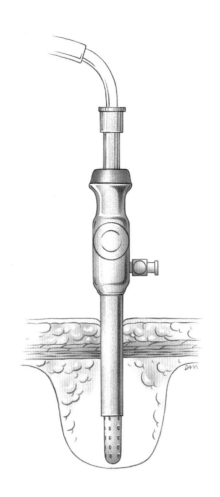

Figure 7.5
The sump suction is passed through a 10 mm port and is used to blindly suck out the fluid, blood or free floating tissue. It is efficient and atraumatic.

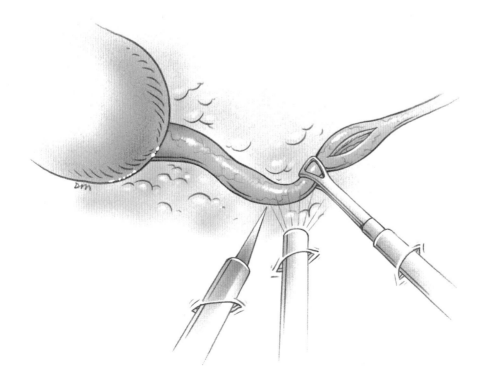

Figure 7.6
The right ureter has been grabbed with an endo-Babcock through the iliac port and pressed over the psoas to make the stone-bearing ureter lie obliquely for easy incision with an endoknife through the posterior port. The kidney is also seen with the camera through the balloon port.

Figure 7.7
The 10 mm cup forceps can fully or partly engulf a stone measuring up to 18 by 12 mm, and can remove it through the 10 mm cannula if fully closed.

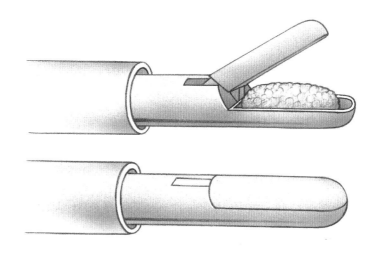

Figure 7.8
The dilated proximal ureter and the pelvicalyceal system are flushed out with a catheter mounted over the tip of a curved 5 mm cannula through the iliac port. Suction is used through the posterior port.

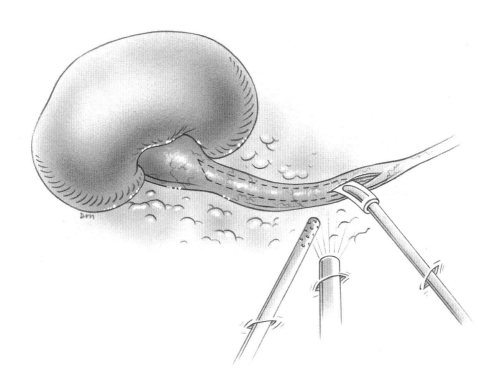

The irrigating fluid is sucked out at the end of the procedure and flushed out stones, if any, are removed.

Ureteral suturing and stenting
During the early part of the surgeon's learning curve, it is better not to suture the ureter, as a badly done job can be responsible for a stricture formation. The postoperative urinary leak can be minimized in these cases by inserting a double-J stent either preoperatively or intraoperatively.

Ureteral suturing is done with 3/0 or 4/0 chromic catgut and the knots can be applied extracorporeally or intracorporeally. Two to three interrupted sutures are usually required to close the ureteral incision. As knot tying can sometimes be difficult and frustrating, the author uses a simple method of clip ligation [11]. After applying a horizontal mattress suture with the end lying extracorporeally, the needle is taken out through the same port. The ureter is lifted up by pulling the two ends of the catgut and a clip is applied close to the serosa (Fig. 7.9). The clip prevents the pursing effect of the mattress suture and assures good apposition of the ureteral edges. Shifting the camara to the iliac position during this manoeuvere makes endoscopic manipulation easier. Fibrin glue suturing of the ureter should be able to offer a much easier alternative [7].

We do not advocate stenting the ureter routinely, as after it has been sutured there is hardly any leak. This also avoids a foreign body reaction and the need to readmit the patient for its removal.

Closure of the ports
The retroperitoneum and the puncture sites are thoroughly checked for any bleeding pints. Blood clots, balloon pieces or washed out stones, if any, are removed and the ureter is properly aligned. A 24F tube drain is passed through the anterior port and is positioned either endoscopically or by digital guidance. All the cannulae are removed and the drain fixed with a cutaneous suture and connected to a drainage bag. The 5 mm port is closed with a single cutaneous suture but the others are closed in layers using 2/0 or 3/0 vicryl. Long-acting local anaesthetic may be infiltrated around the ports for postoperative pain relief.

Iliac approach

The iliac approach to the lower or mid-ureter is very similar to the lumbar approach to the mid-ureter except for the position of the patient and the location of the ports (Fig. 7.10).

A sand bag is placed under the ipsilateral sacroiliac joint of the patient in a supine position. A 2 cm skin incision is made at McBurney's point and is deepened to the external oblique aponeurosis, which is also incised. The retroperitoneal space is exposed by blunt dissection and thereafter a digital dissection is performed to create a space in the retroperitoneum over the psoas

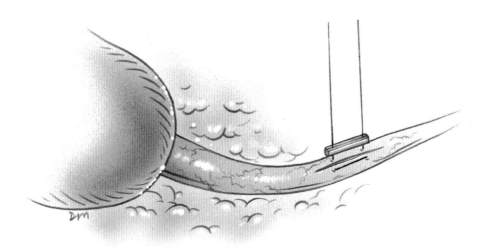

Figure 7.9
The incision in the ureter has been closed by a clip over a mattress suture.

Figure 7.10
Position of the patient and port placement for iliac retroperitoneoscopy: a 10 mm port and the incision for balloon insertion at McBurney's point, a 5 mm port just medial to the anterior superior spine, a 10 mm port about 6 cm above and lateral to the balloon port, and a 10 mm port about 8 cm further up and posteriorly.

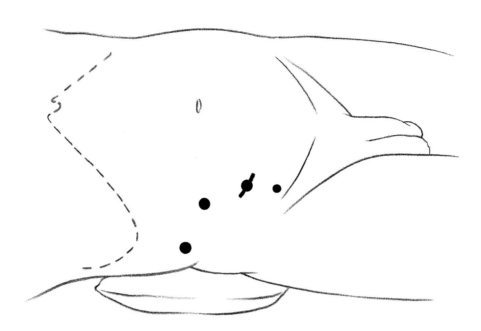

muscle. As the fascia transversalis is thin here, no attempt is made to incise it and the balloon is placed outside the fascia the digitally dissected retroperitoneal space. A 5 mm trocar is placed in the inguinal region medial to the anterior superior spine. Two 10 mm trocars are placed, one about 6 cm cranial and slightly posterior to the balloon port and another about 8 cm posteriorly. This last port is too far away for digital guidance and has to be placed endoscopically. A 0° laparoscope for the mid-ureter or a 30° laparoscope for the lower ureter is used through the iliac or lumbar port. The surgeon uses the inguinal and balloon ports for endoscopic manipulations. The ureter is usually easily identified as it crosses the common iliac artery. The gonadal vessel can be seen anterior to the ureter at this level.

Postoperative care

This is similar to that described in Chapter 6. The patient is discharged with the drain, which is kept until it becomes dry in 2–10 days' time. In most patients a combination of trimethoprim and sulfamethoxazol is continued for the period that the drain or double-J stent is in position.

Clinical experience

Of the 25 reported cases of retroperitoneoscopic ureterolithotomies, 21 were performed at the Bombay Hospital Institute of Medical Sciences [13–20]. All patients had large chronically impacted calculi and were mostly considered for this procedure as an alternative to an open ureterolithotomy, as ESWL and endourological procedures were not available to them. Sixteen patients had upper ureteral calculi, four had mid-ureteral calculi and one had a lower ureteral calculus. The calculi were multiple in only one patient and ranged between 10 and 40 mm in their long axis.

Most procedures were performed using the lumbar approach and the mean operative time was 1 hour without ureteral suturing. Until recently the ureters were left unsutured and most were unstented. Though the patients were discharged the next day, they had to wear the drains under their clothes for up to 10 days. With more experience and the development of the clip suturing technique, we now close all ureteral incisions, which takes less than half an hour, and consequently the drains are removed within 2 days.

Eighteen of our 21 patients had retroperitoneoscopic ureterolithotomies performed successfully and there were no complications. The procedure failed in three patients during the early part of the learning curve due to inexperience and lack of proper instruments; these were converted into open mini operations by joining two of the incisions placed along the kidney incision line.

Conclusion

Retroperitoneoscopic ureteral surgery is a simple, minimally invasive viable alternative to open surgery. Though the whole of the ureter can be easily approached retroperitoneoscopically, the transperitoneal approach provides a better exposure to the lower ureter. A large impacted ureteral calculus has been the commonest indication so far for retroperitoneoscopic exposure of the ureter, either due to non-availability of other minimally invasive modalities or due to their failure to do the job.

References

1   Wickham JEA, The surgical treatment of urolithiasis. In: Wickham JEA, ed. *Urinary Calculus Disease*. New York: Churchill Livingstone, 1979: 145–98.
2   Gaur DD. Laparoscopic operative retroperitoneoscopy: use of a new device. *J Urol* 1992; **148**: 1137–9.
3   Williams PL, Warwick R. Myology. In: Williams PL, Warwick R, eds. *Gray's Anatomy*, 36th edn. Edinburgh: Churchill Livingstone, 1980: 506–93.
4   Clayman RV, Preminger GM, Franklin JR, Curry T, Peters PC. Percutaneous ureterolithotomy. *J Urol* 1985; **133**: 671–4.
5   Meretyk S, Clayman RV, Myers JA. Retroperitoneoscopy: foreign body retrieval. *J Urol* 1992; **147**: 1608–11.
6   Janetschek G, Droxi H, Reissigi A, Bartsch G. Laparoscopic Lich–Gregoir for vesicoureteral reflux (abstract V3-105). *J Endourol* 1994; **8**(Suppl.): S94.
7   Anidjar M, Desgranchamps F, Martin L *et al*. Laparoscopic fibrin glue ureteral anastomosis: an acute experimental study in the porcine model (abstract V1-43A). *J Endourol* 1994: **8**(Suppl.): S55.
8   Gaur DD, Agarwal DK, Purohit KC, Darshane AS. Retroperitoneal laparoscopic pyelolithotomy and pyeloplasty (abstract V-151). *J Endourol* 1993; **7**(Suppl.) S237.
9   Chiu AW, Chen KK, Chang LS. Retroperitoneoscopic dismembered pyeloplasty for ureteropelvic junction obstruction (abstract V4-110). *J Endourol* 1994; **8**(Suppl.): S60.
10 Gaur DD. The use of Hegar's dilator in laparoscopy. *J Min Inv Therapy* 1993; **2**: 33–4.
11 Gaur DD. Retroperitoneal laparoscopy: some technical modifications. *Br J Urol* (in press).
12 Clayman RV. Secondary trocar placement. In Clayman RV, McDougall EM, eds. *Laparoscopic Urology*. St Louis: Quality Medical Publishing, 1993 pp. 66–85.
13 Gaur DD. Retroperitoneal laparoscopic ureteroliyhotomy. *World J Urol* 1993; **11**: 175–8.
14 Harewood LM. Laparoscopic ureterolithotomy; results of an early series. Presented to the BAUS annual meeting, Harrogate, UK, 1993.
15 Gaur DD, Agarwal DK, Purohit KC *et al*. Laparoscopic ureterolithotomy; our experience in 17 patients. *Bombay Hosp J* 1993; **35**: 65.
16 Gaur DD, Purohit KC, Agarwal DK, Darshane AS. Laparoscopic ureterolithootmy for impacted lower ureteral calculi: initial case report. *J Min Inv Therapy* 1993; **2**: 264–6.

17 Gaur DD. Retroperitoneal surgery of the kidney, ureter and adrenal. *Endosc Surg* 1995; **3**: 3–8.
18 Harewood LM, Webb DR, Pope A. Retroperitoneal laparoscopic ureterolithotomy utilizing balloon dilatation of the retroperitoneum (abstract V-160). *J Endourol* 1993; **7**(Suppl.): S239.
19 Rassweiler J, Henkel TO, Stock C *et al*. Retroperitoneoscopy for ablative and reconstructive procedures. Presented to the SIU meeting, Sydney, Australia 1994.
20 Gill IS, Das S, Munch LC. Retroperitoneoscopy; a viable alternative (abstract P4-135). *J Endourol* 1994; **8**(Suppl.): S91.

Chapter 8
Endoscopic subfascial division of incompetent perforating calf veins

P.A. Paraskeva and A.W. Darzi

Introduction

Incompetent perforating veins in the medial compartment of the calf are believed to be a major cause of varicose veins, lipodermatosclerosis and leg ulcers. Cockett, Linton and Boyd originally described the location of these veins connecting the deep venous system to the posterior arch and long saphenous veins, respectively [1,2,3]. Even in the era of duplex Doppler scanning, the management of incompetent calf perforating veins remains a therapeutic challenge. Subfascial or extrafascial ligation, described by Cockett and Linton, have been employed in the management of recurrent perforators with or without lipodermatosclerosis [1,2]. However, these operations have considerable morbidity associated with large incisions through ulcerated areas that heal poorly. We describe a modified technique of endoscopic management of incompetent perforators which does not include an incision in the gaiter area.

Surgical technique

Under general anaesthesia, the patient is placed supine and the whole limb and groin areas are prepared and draped in the usual manner. Through a groin skin crease incision, the saphenofemoral junction is identified, the tributaries ligated and divided, and the long saphenous vein is disconnected from the femoral vein. A stripping device is inserted through the cut end of the long saphenous vein and passed distally where it is retrieved from a small medial incision below the knee. The long saphenous vein is then stripped. Through the same incision below the knee, the fascia lata is exposed and opened between stay sutures. A sterile tourniquet is then placed above the knee and inflated to above arterial pressure after elevation has emptied the limb for several minutes. The subfascial space is developed initially by finger dissection to accept a 10 mm 0° operating endoscope connected to a video endoscopic camera (Storz, Karl Storz, GmbH an & Co, Tuttlingen, Germany) (Fig 8.1) Filmy adhesions between the deep fascia and muscle are broken down with blunt dissection employing the endoscope. To help in creating an operating space in the subfacial compartment the author has adopted the use of a modified size 10.5 endotracheal tube (Portex Medical, Kent, UK) (Fig. 8.2).

Figure 8.1
*Diagram to show the
technique of insertion of the
operating endoscope
surrounded by the modified
10.5 mm endotracheal tube
in to an incision on the
medial side of the knee. Also
shown is the position of the
inflated balloon.*

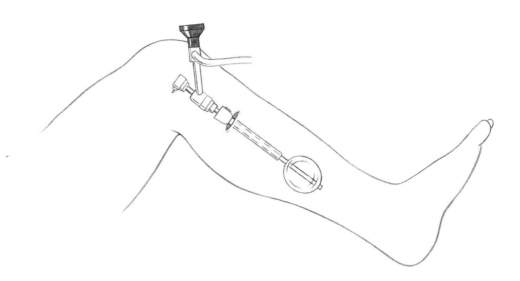

Figure 8.2
*Operating endoscope (Karl
Storz) with a modified
10.5 mm endotracheal tube
(Portex), together with a
syringe to inflate the balloon
on the tube.*

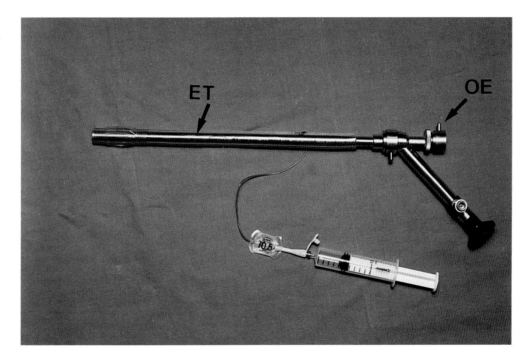

Once inside the subfascial compartment, the cuff of the endotracheal tube is
inflated to create a working space between the fascia and the underlying muscle.
Once the perforating veins are identified, accompanying arteries or nerves, if
present, are carefully dissected off the vein. The veins are then either coagulated
using modified bipolar diathermy graspers (Storz, Karl Storz, GmbH an & Co),
or if the perforating vein is larger than 3 mm then a specially designed loadable
clip applicator is used to clip the vein (Storz, Karl Storz, GmbH an & Co)
(Fig. 8.3). The instruments are passed through an integral operating channel.
The endoscope is then passed distally until all the perforating veins have been
identified. On average, three perforators are identified per patient. In the
presence of lipodermatosclerosis, endoscopic fasciotomy is performed using a

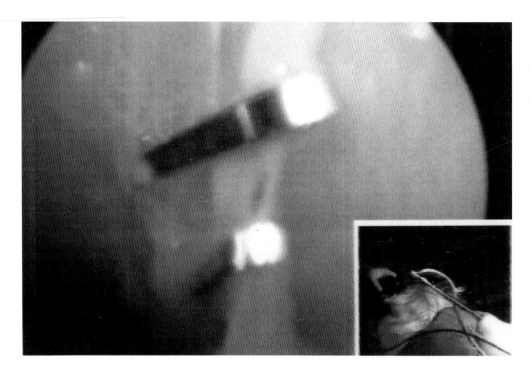

Figure 8.3
Two clips are applied prior to dividing the perforating vein. The insert shows the operating endoscope with the overlying endotrachael tube inserted through the incision below the knee.

hook knife (Storz, Karl Storz, GmbH an & Co) (Fig. 8.4). At the end of the procedure the groin and below knee incisions are closed and the limb is bandaged.

Discussion

Although incompetent perforating veins can be identified at open surgery, their detection is blind and is associated with multiple, painful and sometimes cosmetically undesirable scars. The endoscopic approach allows identification of perforators by direct vision with accurate division, and avoids multiple stab incisions. The use of the endoscopic technique in combination with a high saphenous ligation may be useful in both primary and particularly recurrent varicose veins [4–7].

Endoscopic surgery for incompetent perforating veins may also provide new options for the management of venous ulcers. Effective operations for venous ulcers that involve subfascial ligation of veins have shown some efficacy [1,2] but the problems with these procedures are that large incisions and extensive dissections are required, which lead to a high postoperative morbidity with incisions made through poor quality tissues showing trophic changes. By using an endoscopic approach these problems can be avoided.

The technique of endoscopic subfascial ligation of incompetent perforating veins has been used with great effect in Europe, although experience is still limited and complications such as subfascial haematoma and tibial nerve damage have been reported [4,7]. Hauer and co-workers were the first to describe an endoscopic approach in the management of incompetent perforating veins in the calf [4,5]. Subsequently, Fischer described in a similar approach employing a modified sigmoidoscope where the veins were coagulated using diathermy [6,7]. However, these approaches have the disadvantages of having a small field of

Figure 8.4
The fasciotomy hook knife divides the fascia lata. The insert is as in Fig. 8.2.

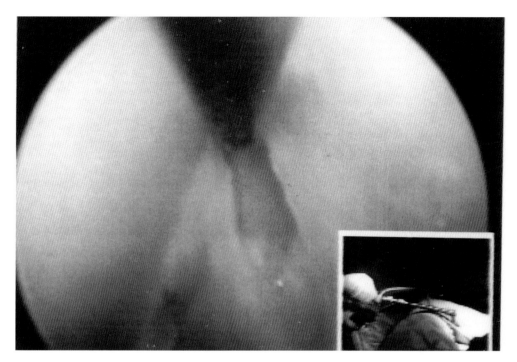

vision, where the manipulation of the instruments and the identification of the perforators is difficult. The modified endotracheal tube greatly facilitates space creation, especially in areas of lipodermatosclerosis where the subfascial space is very tight. In addition, this method allows tenting of the perforating veins as they cross the fascia lata, facilitating their accurate division.

In conclusion, early results of endoscopic subfascial ligation of perforating veins are promising. However, as with most other minimal access procedures this approach requires further critical evaluation especially with regard to its potential in the management of recurrent varicose veins and venous ulceration.

References

1   Cockett FB. The pathology and treatment of venous ulcers of the leg. *Br J Surg* 1955; **43**: 260–78.
2   Linton RR. The communicating veins of the lower leg and operative techniques for their ligation. *Ann Surg* 1938; **107**: 582–93.
3   Boyd AM. Treatment of varicose veins. *Proc R Soc Med* 1961; **41**: 633–9.
4   Hauer G. Operationstechnik der endoskopischen subfascialen discision der perforansvenen. *Chirurgie* 1987; **58**: 172–5.
5   Hauer G, Borkun J, Wigger I, Diller S. Endoscopic subfascial dissection of perforating veins. *Surg Endosc* 1988; **2**: 5–12.
6   Fischer RH. Diagnosis and treatment of incompetent Cokett perforators veins by endoscopy: present state. In: Raymond-Martibeau P, Prescott R, Zummo M, eds. *Phlebologie 92*. Paris: John Libbey Eurotext, 1992: 1086.
7   Fischer R. Erfahrungen mit der endoskopischen perforantensanierung. *Phlebologie* 1992; **21**: 224–9.

Chapter 9

Laparoscopic groin hernia repair

J-L. Dulucq

Introduction

Laparoscopic treatment of inguinal hernias represents a step forward, in view of the increased comfort and benefit for the patient. The technique presented in this chapter consists of treating a hernia with the placement of a Prolene (60/110 or 85/120) mesh between the muscle wall and the peritoneal sack. Using mesh for hernia repair is of the utmost importance for subsequent robustness. The introduction and positioning of the mesh are perfromed laparoscopically, after the creation of a pre- and retropneumoperitoneum.

This strictly extraperitoneal technique is another implementation of minimally invasive endoscopic surgery. Professor Stoppa's work [1,2] has proved that pre- and retroperitoneal mesh placement is reliable as well as being well tolerated, by the patient. The laparoscopic approach of the retroperitoneal space, performed in a standardized way, currently appears to be fully satisfactory.

Indications

Originally, only medium-sized external oblique hernias on male patients were treated. We currently treat external oblique hernias associated with a direct component, direct hernias, bilateral inguinal hernias, medium-sized inguinoscrotal hernias and hernia recurrences. As a rule we only refuse voluminous inguinoscrotal hernias. Previous subumbilical laparotomy is not a contraindication to this approach, but tends to make it more difficult.

Special care must be taken in trocar positioning. The retropneumoperitoneum is always well tolerated, and contraindications are the same as in conventional surgery.

Preoperative check

The preoperative check is the same as in conventional surgery, using standard blood tests, a lung X-ray and an cardiovascular check up. Parietal ultrasonography may also be prescribed in particular cases.

Surgical technique

Equipment

1 Imagery:
  one video monitor,
  one 450 W xenon light source,
  one video camera,
  one 10 mm laparoscope, 0°,
  one 10 mm laparoscope, 30°,
  one U-matic video recorder.

2 Instrumentation (Fig. 9.1)
  two 10 mm trocars,
  one 5 mm trocar,
  one reducer,
  one palpator,
  two grasping forceps,
  one scissor,
  one automatic clip applier.

3 Creation of the pneumoperitoneum:
  6 l/min insufflation,
  one veress needle.

Figure 9.1
Instruments.

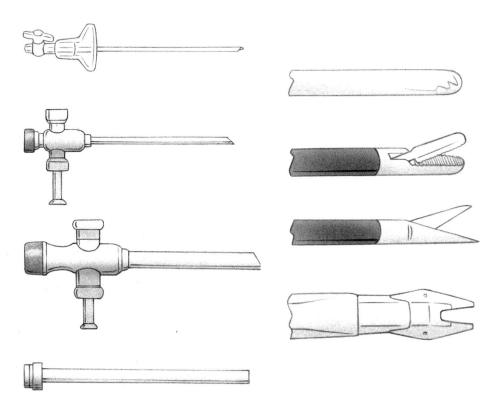

Position of the patient

The patient, placed under general anaesthesia through tracheal intubation or, more rarely, under peridural anaesthesia, lies supine on the operating table (Fig. 9.2). A urinary catheter is inserted. The operating table has a 10% reversed Trendelenburg position available. The surgeon stands on the opposite side from the hernia. The assistant faces the surgeon slightly obliquely, and the scrub nurse stands by his or her side.

Creation of the retropneumoperitoneum

Before inserting the main trocar, 1 litre of carbon dioxide (CO_2) is insufflated in to the Retzius space through suprapubical direct perforation with a Veress needle. The needle must be positioned through the aponeurosis and behind it, in the virtual space represented by the Retzius space. The maximum pressure setting for the insufflator is 10 mmHg. This preliminary dissection of the subperitoneal space will allow easy insertion of the first trocar without any risk of peritoneal puncture.

Trocar placement

Three trocars are needed (Fig. 9.3):

1 One 10 mm trocar on the inferior margin of the umbilicus.
2 One 5 mm trocar inserted suprapubically on the median line, two fingers above the pubis.
3 One 10 mm trocar inserted vertically from the upper anterior iliac spine.

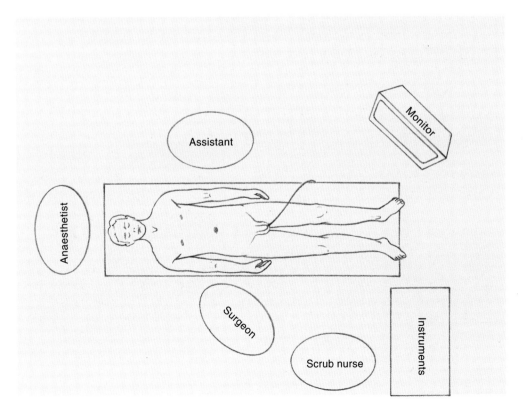

Figure 9.2
Position of the patient and position of the surgeon.

Figure 9.3
Display of trocars.

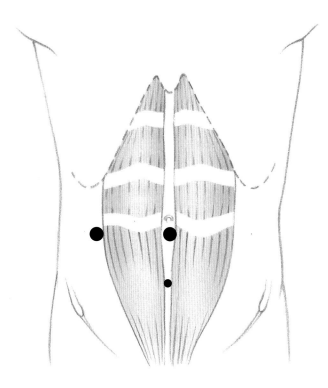

The first trocar, together with its mandrin, is first introduced subcutaneously below the inferior margin of the umbilicus to a depth of 5 mm. The trocar then crosses the aponeurosis tangentially, before reaching the subperitoneal space created by CO_2 insufflation through the Veress needle.

Instrumentation layout

The following instruments are introduced successively: the optical system in the first trocar, the E palpator in the second trocar, one F grasping forceps in the third trocar after placement of the D reducer, then the H automatic clip applier is introduced through the third trocar.

Exposition of the main anatomical landmarks (Fig. 9.4)

A blunt mandrin is introduced through the 5 mm second trocar which allows the dissection of the peritoneal sac to be continued and the exposure of the first anatomical landmark — the Cooper ligament. Once the Cooper ligament has been discovered, all the other anatomical components should be easily located. The second anatomical landmark, the epigastric pedicle located in the roof of the dissecting field, may be difficult to locate if a direct inguinal hernia is found (whose reduction is necessary and always easy to complete). Dissection of the epigastric pedicle reveals the upper edge of the hernia sac.

Skeletonization of the hernia sac (Fig. 9.5 and 9.6)

On the lower edge of the epigastric pedicle, the upper edge of the peritoneal sac is dissected and lowered gradually, thanks to the E palpator. On the outside, and

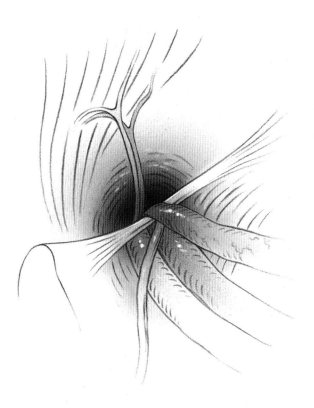

Figure 9.4
Exposition of the main anatomical landmarks.

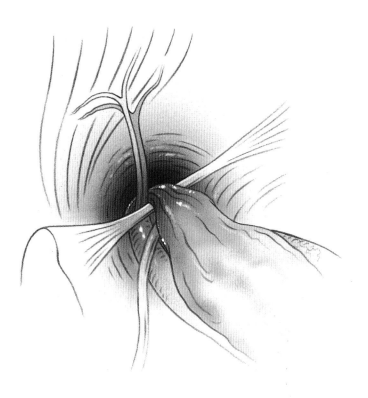

Figure 9.5
Exposition of the hernia sac.

Figure 9.6
Dissection of the hernia sac.

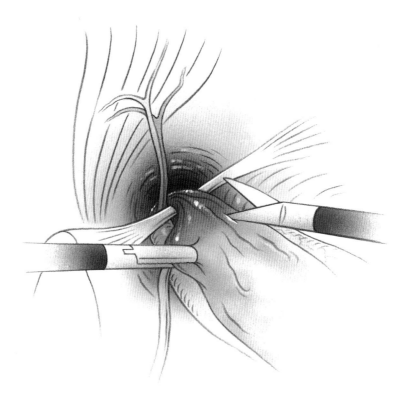

beyond this limit, the palpator proceeds more quickly due to the lower resistance of the peritoneal attachments. Skeletonization of the peritoneal sac is thus completed, and the third 10–11 mm trocar with reducer 5 is inserted level with the iliac fossa, opposite the anterior superior iliac spine.

Introduction of an F grasping forceps through this trocar will allow the skeletonization of the peritoneal sac to be completed through dissection of the psoas muscle fibres. Two instruments are now ready and dissection of the hernia sac can proceed.

Dissection of the peritoneal sac and parietalization of the cord elements
(Fig. 9.7)

The G microscissors are inserted through the second orifice. The hernia sac can now be dissected gradually and freed from the inguinal orifice. It is then put aside in the abdominal cavity, and the elements of the spermatic cord, the spermatic vessels and the vas deferens are progressively dissected, freed from the peritoneum and thus parietalized as high as possible in the abdominal cavity. Lastly, thanks to the F grasping forceps introduced through the second and third trocars, the various neighbouring anatomical components can be dissected completely. The Cooper ligament is fully exposed. The iliac vessels are located and the spermatic cord is freed completely from the peritoneal bag. The psoas muscle is dissected and, finally, the peritoneal sac is pushed up as far high as possible in the abdominal cavity.

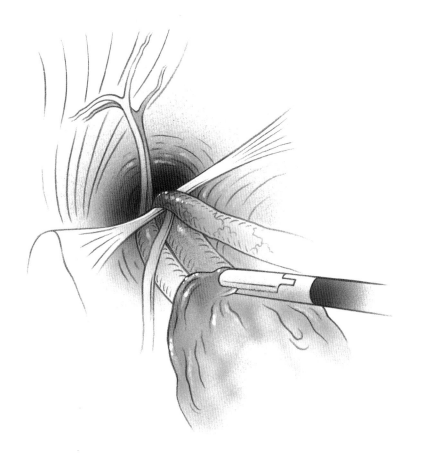

Figure 9.7
Dissection of the peritoneal sac.

Placement and fastening of the mesh (Fig. 9.8)

The 80/130 mm Prolene mesh is first rolled up and then introduced through the third trocar in the iliac fossa. Once inside, it is positioned in front of the inguinal orifices. Its shape is that of a curved tile. Its lower edge is fastened to the Cooper ligament and to the most external part of the psoas muslce; this is done under visual control to avoid nerve injury. The fastening is done with two titanium clips applied with the H automatic clip applier introduced through the third trocar. The lower edge of the prothesis thus bridges the iliac vessels and the elements of the spermatic cord parietalized posteriorly. The mesh is then applied to the external inguinal orifice; its upper edge will cling to the wall when it changes shape during exsufflation of the retropneumoperitoneum. The pneumoperitoneum is slowly evacuated at the end of the procedure and no drainage is installed.

Specific problems of the method

The key to this operation is the creation of the retropneumoperitoneum. It begins with preliminary suprapubic insufflation of 1 litre of CO_2, which initiates subperitoneal detachment. The next step is the skeletonization of the sac. Respect of the various sequences guarantees the reliability of the method, but several incidents have been observed:

Figure 9.8
Placement and fastening of the mesh.

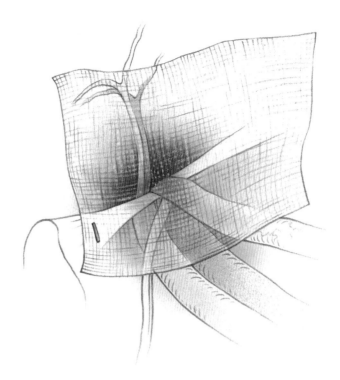

1 Subcutaneous emphysema of medium extent, due to the retropneumoperitoneum, near the puncture sites. The trocars should be inserted with extreme care.
2 Minor scrotal emphysema, easily evacuated by simple pressure at the end of the procedure.
3 Haematomata near the external inguinal orifice, which were drained by simple puncture, with no recurrence.
4 Breaking into the peritoneum during the procedure does not mean that the peritoneum should be interrupted. It is, however, necessary to balance the intraperitoneal and extraperitoneal pressures. If the peritoneal defect is only a small hole, and intraperitoneal trocar acting as a safety valve should be inserted.

Clinical experience

From June 1990 to June 1995, 864 inguinal hernias in 797 patients were treated using the method described in this chapter. There were 462 external oblique inguinal hernias, 272 direct inguinal hernias, 71 direct hernias combined with an external oblique inguinal hernia, 67 bilateral inguinal hernias and 70 recurrent hernias. All patients were checked 1 month and 3 months postoperatively. The results were excellent, characterized by extreme robustness and a high degree of reliability. The average hospital stay was 48–72 hours. Early in our experience we had eight conversions to traditional surgery and two conversions to laparoscopic transperitoneal surgery.

Complications included the following:

1 Twenty-six cases of minor subcutaneous emphysema.
2 Twenty-four cases of haematomata of the external inguinal orifice, two of which had to be drained surgically.

There were:

1 Eight immediate re-operations; seven through laparoscopy and one through open surgery.
2 Three immediate recurrences due to inadequate positioning of the mesh and spontaneous folding of its upper edge.
3 Three laparoscopic re-operations for acute pain in the crural nerve area, demanding immediate removal of the ill-positioned clip fastening the mesh to the psoas muscle.
4 Two immediate laparoscopic re-operations to evacuate a very large haematoma in front of the mesh. These were not followed by drainage.

These last five re-operations took place at day 2 postoperatively and there were no recurrences.

Discussion

The laparoscopic approach for the treatment of inguinal hernias is quite appropriate. It reduces aponeurosis of the muscle and skin deterioration linked with conventional surgical treatment. We opted for the retroperitoneal route as early as June 1990. In view of open surgery achievements for this same approach, the laparoscopic retroperitoneal procedure appears to be the most logical and most reliable one in the long run. McKernan and Phillips [3–5] and Begin [6–9] followed close in our tracks, with a very similar approach.

Laparoscopic techniques using the transperitoneal route seem to be less successful because of possible adhesions, post-operative pain due to the pneumoperitoneum and postoperative bowel obstruction. Finally, the difficulties frequently encountered in achieving a proper closure of the peritoneal sac seem to be greater [10,11].

Simple intraperitoneal clipping on of the mesh without peritoneal protection seems to be even less in keeping with the necessarily harmless character of inguinal hernia treatment. The mesh, made of Prolene (an inert semirigid material), seems well suited to the retroperitoneal space under laparoscopy. It is well tolerated but it must be fastened so as to avoid immediate postoperative shifting.

Conclusion

The increasing use of this technique and its reliability in the creation of the pneumoperitoneum has meant that hernia repair through retroperitoneoscopy is now a promising implementation of minimally-invasive laparoscopic surgery. This simple and efficient method is able to achieve perfect results.

References

1 Stoppa RE, Warlaumont CR. The preperitoneal approach and prosthetic repair of groin hernia. In : Nyphus LM, Condon RE, eds, Hernia. Philadelphia: *JP lippincottm*, 1989: 199–255.
2 Stoppa RE, Rives JL, Warlaumont CR. The use of Dacron in the repair of hernias of the groin. *Surg Clin N Am* 1984; **64**: 269–85.
3 McKernan JB, Laws HL. Laparoscopic repair of inguinal hernias using a totally extraperitoneal prosthetic approach. *Surg Endosc* 1993; **7**: 26–8.

4   Philips EH, Caroll BJ, Pearlstein AR, Daykhovsky L, Fallas MJ. Laparoscopic choledochoscopy and extraction of common bile duct stones. *World J Surg* 1993; **17**: 22–8

5   Philips EH, Franklin M, Carroll BJ *et al.* Laparoscopic colectomy. Ann Surg 1992; **216**: 703–7.

6   Begin G. *Surg Endosc* 1992; **6**(4).

7   Begin G. *J Coelio-Chir* 1993; 8.

8   Begin G. *Chir Endosc* 1992; 1.

9   Begin G. *J Laparoendosc Surg* 1990; **1**(1).

10 Fitzgibbons RJ Jr, Annibali R, Litke BS. Gallbladder and gallstone removal, open versus closed laparoscopy, and pneumoperitoneum. *Am J Surg* 1993; **165**: 497–504.

11 Fitzgibbons RJ Jr. Laparoscopic hernia repair. In: *Proceedings of Symposium on New Frontiers in Endosurgery.* New Brunswick, NJ: Ethicon Inc, 1991.

Further reading

Arregui M, Devis C, Yucel O, Nagan R. Laparoscopic mesh repair of inguinal hernia using a preperitoneal approach: a preliminary report. *Surg Laparosc Endosc* 1992; **2**: 53–8.

Corbitt JD Jr. Laparoscopic herniorrhaphy. *Surg Laparosc Endosc* 1991; **1**: 23–5.

Dulucq JL. Traitement des hernies de l'aine par mise en place d'un patch prothétique sous-péritonéal en rétropéritonéoscopie. *Cah Chir* 1991; **79**: 15–16.

Dulucq JL. Traitment of inguinal hernias by insertions of mesh through retroperitoneoscopy. *Postgrad Gen Surg* 1992; **4**(2): 173–4.

Ferzli G, Raboy A, Kleinerman D, Albert P. Extraperitoneal endoscopic pelvic lymph node dissection vs. laparoscopic lymph node dissection in the staging of prostatic and bladder carcinoma. *J Laparoendosc Surg* 1992; **2**: 219–22.

Himpens J. Laparoscopic hernioplasty using a self-expandable (umbrella-like) prosthetic patch. *Surg Laparosc Endosc* 1992; **2**(4): 312–16.

Himpens J. Laparoscopic inguinal hernioplasty: repair with a conventional vs a new self-expandable mesh. *Surg Endosc* 1993: **7**: 315–19.

Lichtenstein IL, Shulman AJ, Amid PK *et al.* The tension-free hernioplasty. *Am J Surg* 1989; **157**: 188–93.

Toy FK, Smoot RT. Toy Smoot hernioplasty. *Surg Laparosc Endosc* 1991; **1**: 151–5.

Vernay A. La rétropéritonéoscopie: justification anatomique. Expérimentation technique. Expérience clinique. Thèse Medical Grenoble, 1980.

Webb DR, Redgrave N, Chan Y, Harewood LM. Extraperitoneal laparoscopy: early experience and evaluation. *Aust N Z J Surg* 1993; **63**: 554–7.

Wurtz A. L'endoscopie de l'espace rétropéritonéal: techniques, résultats et indications actuelles. *Ann Chir* 1989; **43**: 475–80.

Chapter 10

Retroperitoneal approaches to the aorta and its branches

H.H. Sigurdsson and P.A. Grace

Introduction

The incidence of abdominal aortic aneurysms is continuing to rise [1,2] and as the proportion of the population aged over 65 years increases [3], aneurysmal and occlusive aortic disease will continue to be a major source of mortality and morbidity in the elderly [4,5]. Screening programmes may identify patients with asymptomatic aneurysms suitable for elective surgical repair, a procedure that now carries a mortality of less than 5% [6–8]. Transabdominal aortic endoaneurysmorraphy with graft replacement, as evolved by Creech [9], is now the generally accepted and most widely applied surgical approach to infrarenal abdominal aortic aneurysms [7,10,11]. However, it has been recognized for many years that the aorta can be approached by the retroperitoneal route with a significant reduction in operative morbidity and hospitalization [12,13]. The purpose of this chapter is to review the impact of the retroperitoneal exposure of the infrarenal abdominal aorta and its branches in the management of patients with aneurysmal or occlusive aortoiliac disease. Other indications for retroperitoneal dissection are listed in Table 10.1. However, apart from the vascular operations, these procedures will not be discussed further in this chapter.

History of retroperitoneal exposure in arterial surgery

John Abernathy first described a retroperitoneal dissection when in 1796 he tried, unsuccessfully, to ligate an external iliac artery aneurysm [14]. In 1834, Murray, in South Africa, reported a case of ligature of the abdomina aorta and commented that the operation was more tedious than difficult and at one time the patient needed some brandy and water to support him! Unfortunately, in spite of the brandy, the patient died 23 hours after the operation [15]. Sir Astley Cooper used the retroperitoneal approach 2 years later to ligate the external iliac artery in a patient with femoral aneurysm [16].

The first modern resection of an abdominal aortic aneurysm was performed in 1951 by Dubost, Allary and Oeconomos, who gained access to the aorta extraperitoneally via a left thoracoabdominal incision [17]. Rob, in 1963, reported 500 cases of aortic reconstruction in which he used the retroperitoneal route and observed a better postoperative course in these patients compared with patients undergoing transperitoneal aneurysm repair [12]. However, he cautioned against the retroperitoneal route in patients with large aneurysms or aneurysms which

Table 10.1
*Common retroperitoneal
operations.*

Vascular	Aortic or iliac aneurysm repair
	Aortofemoral bypass
	Aortoiliac bypass
	Aortorenal or iliorenal bypass
	Aortopopliteal or iliopopliteal bypass
	Coeliac or mesenteric endarterectomy/angioplasty/bypass
	Lumbar sympathectomy
	Renal artery endarterectomy/angioplasty/bypass
Urological	Lymphadenectomy for testicular cancer
	Nephrectomy
	Nephroureterectomy
	Pyeloplasty
	Reimplantation of ureters
	Renal cyst resection
	Ureterolithotomy
	Ureterolysis
Endocrine	Adrenalectomy
Orthopaedic	Anterior spinal fusion
Transplant	Renal transplantation

extended to the juxtarenal level. Although impressed with the decreased morbidity associated with the procedure, he commented that retraction was difficult. This may have been because of poor patient positioning and an inadequate incision [12]. Rob also noted that ruptured aneurysms could be satisfactorily excised via the retroperitoneal approach and that the extravasated blood had dissected the retroperitoneum in many cases.

In the succeeding 20 years the retroperitoneal technique was championed by Stipa and Shaw [18], Helsby and Moossa [19] and Stoney and Wylie [20], who approached thoracoabdominal aneurysms via a transpleural chest incision extending across the costal margin into the true retroperitoneal space from the left side. More recently, Taheri *et al.* [21], Williams *et al.* [22], Sharp and Donavan [13], Corson *et al.* [23] and Leather *et al.* [24] have all reported their experiences with the retroperitoneal approach and have all observed improved morbidity following this technique. In 1994, Rosenbaum and colleages successfully performed retroperitoneal dissection under epidural anaesthesia, thereby further reducing morbidity and patient discomfort and facilitating early hospital discharge [25]. Shepard *et al.* [26] advocated the retroperitoneal approach for high risk abdominal aortic aneurysms in 1986, and in 1988 Chang and his colleagues reported nine patients with ruptured aneurysms in whom repair was achieved via the retroperitoneal route [27].

Technical considerations

A number of different incisions have been described for the retroperitoneal exposure of the aorta and its branches.

1 A midline extraperitoneal incision [28].
2 A left iliac fossa incision [12].
3 A cresentic left paramedian incision only [19,21] or with an oblique extension onto the left anterior chest wall (the Risberg incision) [29] (Fig. 10.1)
4 A transverse left upper abdominal incision [30].
5 Various flank incisions [13,22,24,26,27,31–33] (Fig. 10.2).

The left iliac artery, aortic bifurcation and distal aorta can also be approached retroperitoneally by vertically extending a longitudinal inguinal incision cephalad onto the abdominal wall to the level of the umbilicus — the Peter Martin approach [34,35].

The proponents of the paramedian incisions have observed less postoperative pain compared with flank incisions, presumably because there is less dissection of muscle posteriorly. Risberg's extension of the paramedian incision gives excellent access to the suprarenal aorta [29].

Currently, an oblique flank incision is favoured by most surgeons for retroperitoneal exposure of the aorta [13,22,24,26,27,31,32]. The incision extends in a curvilinear fashion from the lateral border of the rectus muscle at the level of the umbilicus anteriorly to the 11th interspace posteriorly. Using electrocautery, the incision is deepened posteriorly through the lower fibres of

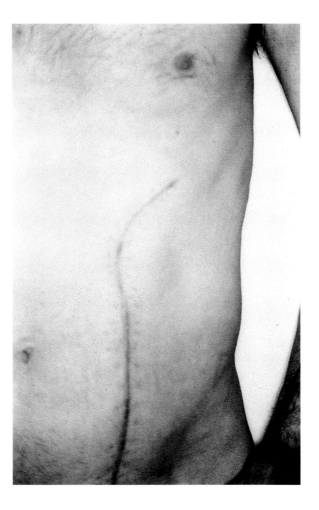

Figure 10.1
The Risberg incision for exposure of the retroperitoneal aorta. The incision is a left cresentic paramedian incision with an extension onto the left anterior chest wall.

Figure 10.2
*A flank incision to gain access
to the retroperitoneal space.
The incision extends from the
lateral border of the rectus
anteriorly to the 11th
interspace posteriorly.*

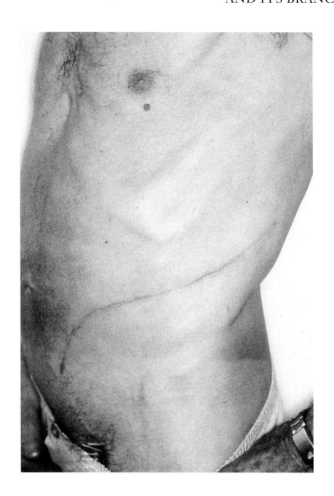

the latissimus dorsi and the underlying edge of the serratus posterior inferior and anteriorly through the external and internal oblique muscles. The lumbar fascia is incised posteriorly to expose the loose fat of the retroperitoneal space. Using blunt dissection, the peritoneum is separated from the posterior surface of the transversus abdominis, which is then divided.

The retroperitoneal space is initially developed inferiorly by blunt finger dissection separating the posterior peritoneum from the iliopsoas muscle taking care to stay anterior to the epimysium of the iliopsoas muscle. This manoeuvre exposes the left external and common iliac arteries and the aorta just above the bifurcation (Fig. 10.3). The dissection then proceeds cephalad, developing the plane between the iliopsoas muscle and the perirenal fascia with its enclosed fat. Most authors advocate mobilization and medial displacement of the left kidney and ureter [24,26,27]. When dealing with an infrarenal aneurysm, however, Sicard *et al.* prefer to leave the kidney in its anatomical position and dissect the left ureter off the peritoneum and retract it laterally to prevent traction injury [31,32]. The left renal artery is easily identified by a line dropped vertically from the tip of the 11th rib.

After systemic heparinization, the iliac arteries should be controlled initially to minimize the potential for distal embolization [24]. This can usually be achieved by lifting the artery forward with a Babcock forceps and applying a shod Fogarty clamp. If difficulty is encountered in placing an external clamp on the right iliac artery, control can be achieved later by balloon intraluminal catheter occlusion,

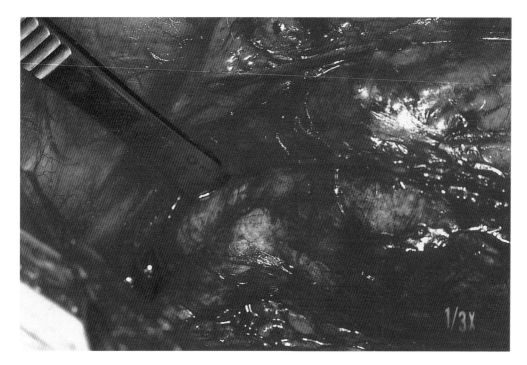

Figure 10.3
Retroperitoneal exposure of the lower aorta and both common iliac arteries in a patient with a small aortic and bilateral common iliac artery aneurysms.

after opening the aneurysm sac. The neck of the aneurysm is approached from its posterolateral aspect. The large lumbar branch of the left renal vein is identified, transfixed and divided. The plane posterior to the neck of the aneurysm is developed by blunt dissection close to the vertebral body. The anterior plane is similarly opened so that a straight shod Fogarty clamp can be applied. No attempt is made to dissect the aorta free circumferentially.

When supracoeliac control is necessary, the dissection proceeds cephalad along the aorta towards the left crus of the diaphragm which is divided along the long axis of the aorta [26]. When approaching a ruptured aneurysm by the retroperitoneal route a hand is inserted along the diaphragm until the crus and underlying supracoeliac aorta are encountered. Manual pressure is applied to the aorta with the left hand while with the right hand the crus is divided transversely immediately caudal to the area of compression and an aortic clamp is applied [27]. The retroperitoneal space is then opened as for an elective aneurysm and the supracoeliac clamp removed [27]. Although most surgeons open the aneurysm sac longitudinally along its posterolateral wall and insert a tube or bifurcated graft using the Creech technique [26,31,32,36], Leather *et al.* prefer to exclude the aneurysm and perform an end-to-end anastomosis between the divided proximal and distal aorta and the graft [24]. The aneurysm sac is then oversewn to exclude it. These authors have argued that this technique reduces blood loss by 40–50% compared with opening the aneurysm sac [24].

After the aneurysm sac is opened, back bleeding from the lumbar and inferior mesenteric arteries is controlled by suture ligation, and the upper anastomosis is performed in the standard fashion. Whenever possible a tube graft should be inserted as this obviates the need to expose the femoral or external iliac arteries. However, in patients with iliac aneurysms or iliac occlusive disease, distal anastomoses are carried out to the iliac or femoral arteries as necessary. The right limb of a bifurcated graft can be easily passed in a retroureteric fashion into the right iliac or right femoral area [31,32]. Shepard *et al.* advocate anastomosing the distal limbs of a bifurcated graft to the external iliac arteries as it is easier and avoids the complications of a groin incision. This is achieved on the left side through the retroperitoneal incision and on the right through a small right lower quadrant incision [26].

Most commonly, the retroperitoneal vascular structures are approached from the left side, however a right retroperitoneal approach using a flank incision best lends itself to a right iliofemoral endarterectomy or right renal artery revascularization (either an aortorenal or an iliorenal bypass.) It can also be used in selected cases of infrarenal aortic aneurysm or aortobifemoral bypass for occlusive disease, particularly if right renal artery revascularization is required. It is also an alternative exposure for patients who have had previous surgery in the left retroperitoneum (i.e. a nephrectomy or sigmoid colectomy). Unlike the left approach, the right retroperitoneal approach is not suitable for coeliac and superior mesenteric revascularization or for repair of juxtarenal or suprarenal aortic aneurysms [33].

Indications

The most frequent indication for the retroperitoneal approach is the elective repair of an infrarenal abdominal aortic aneurysm [22–24]. It is especially useful in patients with high risk aneurysms [26,32]. Shepard *et al.* used the retroperitoneal approach in 23 patients who had either anatomically complex aneurysms ($n = 19$) or were medically high risk patients ($n = 9$) or both ($n = 14$). Three of them had undergone previous abortive attempts at aneurysm repair via the transperitoneal route. There was a single postoperative death (4%) in this high risk group of patients [26]. Sicard *et al.* used the retroperitoneal route for aneurysm repair in 21 high risk patients (American Society of Anaesthesiologists anaesthesia risk classification IV) with a single death and an average postoperative hospital stay of 24 days. These patients, who had significant chronic pulmonary disease, recent (i.e. within 3 months) myocardial infarction, congestive cardiac failure or significant arrhythmias, would not have been considered for aneurysm repair by the transperitoneal route [32].

Ruptured abdominal aortic aneurysms have also been approached via the retroperitoneal route, and Rob in 1963 commented that ruptured aneurysms could be satisfactorily excised via this approach and that in many cases the extravasated blood will have dissected the peritoneum allowing for rapid clamping of the aorta [12]. Chang *et al.*, using an oblique flank incision, reported the use of left retroperitoneal aortic exposure in ruptured ($n = 9$) or symptomatic ($n = 16$) abdominal aortic aneurysms [27]. Without exposing the aneurysm, a hand was inserted along the diaphragm until the crus and underlying supracoeliac aorta were encountered and manual pressure was applied, compressing the aorta against the vertebral column. Manual control could be gained reliably within 5 minutes of intubation. An additional 1–2 minutes was required to place a clamp on the supracoeliac aorta. They had four deaths (16%), one in the rupture group (11%) and three in the symptomatic group (19%). All other patients regained intestinal function within 2 days of operation and all appeared to do better than previous patients with transperitoneal emergency surgery in terms of intensive care and length of hospital stay [27]. The retroperitoneal route has also been used to gain access for juxtarenal and suprarenal aneurysms [32].

Aortoiliac occlusive disease is the other main indication for the retroperitoneal approach to the abdominal aorta and iliac arteries. It has been used extensively for aortoiliac disobliteration [19], aortoiliac bypass, aortofemoral bypass, iliopopliteal bypass, coeliac, mesenteric and renal artery endarterectomy, and angioplasty or bypass of occlusive disease [30,32,37,38]. Metz and Mathiesen reported their experience of the retroperitoneal approach for aortoiliac disease in 52 patients and observed decreased mortality and morbidity compared with the transperitoneal approach in 17 patients [30].

Johnson *et al.* used the extraperitoneal route in the management of 298 patients with claudication ($n = 189$) or critical ischaemia ($n = 109$) [39]. Of these patients, 106 underwent thromboendarterectomy and 192 had a graft inserted. The 30-day mortality rates for claudication and limb salvage were 1.6 and 8.3%, respectively, with significant improvement in morbidity (38 vs 49%) compared with 161 comparable patients treated by the transperitoneal route. However, the mortality rate was 4% for both groups of patients [39]. Mills *et al.* [40] used the retroperitoneal, left flank approach to the supracoeliac aorta to use it as an inflow source for difficult and repeat aortic reconstructions in 11 patients with relative or absolute contraindications to standard infrarenal reconstructions. Indications included multiple failed infrarenal reconstruction ($n = 4$), previous removal of an infected aortobifemoral bypass graft with failure of an extra-anatomic bypass ($n = 5$), prior para-aortic lymph node dissection and radiotherapy ($n = 1$) and aortic aneurysmal disease proximal to the renal arteries ($n = 1$). Using this method the supracoeliac artery can easily be approached without thoracotomy and avoids a difficult infrarenal aortic dissection in a scarred field. In addition, this bypass is likely to be more durable than inflow reconstructions based on the axillary artery. The mean supracoeliac cross clamping time was 24 minutes and only one patient suffered transient postoperative acute tubular necrosis. There was no mortality [40].

Advantages and disadvantages

The earliest proponents of retroperitoneal approaches to the aorta observed that it led to a smoother, less eventful postoperative course with a low incidence of pulmonary complications and ileus [12,18,21,25,28,30,36,37]. To date, however, only two prospective randomized studies comparing the reproperitoneal and transabdominal approaches to the abdominal aorta have been reported [41,42]. Cambria *et al.* randomized 113 patients undergoing elective abdominal aortic reconstruction to transabdominal ($n = 59$) or anterolateral retroperitoneal ($n = 54$) approaches. They were unable to demonstrate statistically any important differences between the two approaches [41]. However, Sicard *et al.* [42] randomized 145 patients undergoing routine surgery for abdominal aortic aneurysm or aortoiliac occlusive disease to transabdominal ($n = 75$) or retroperitoneal ($n = 75$) approaches. They reported that the retroperitoneal approach was associated with fewer postoperative complications (17 (24%) vs 38 (52%)) ($P < 0.0001$), shorter stays in hospital (9.9 ± 2.3 vs 12.9 ± 9.0 days) ($P = 0.10$) and the intensive care unit (2.3 ± 2.3 vs 3.5 ± 4.6 days) ($P = 0.006$), lower incidence of postoperative ileus (0 (0%) vs 8 (11%)) ($P = 0.005$) and lower costs (US $16 350 ± $8746 vs $21 023 ± $14 801) ($P = 0.017$) (Table 10.2).

A number of other authors have also compared the two approaches, but the patients in the transperitoneal groups were either historical controls [30] or

Table 10.2
Comparison of the retroperitoneal and transperitoneal approaches to the aorta.

Study	Retroperitoneal approach					Transperitoneal approach				
	n	Mortality	Morbidity	In-patient days	Ileus	n	Mortality	Morbidity	In-patient days	Ileus
Metz & Mathiesen [30]	52	5 (10%)	27 (52%)	15	3 (6%)	17	2 (12%)	10 (59%)	23	6 (35%)
Johnson et al. [39]	298	12 (4%)	112 (38%)	12	3 (1%)	161	6 (4%)	79 (49%)	17	10 (6%)
Sicard et al. [32]	115	0	–	10	–	98	3 (3%)	–	14	–
Leather et al. [24]	193	7 (4%)	14 (7%)	7	1 (0.5%)	106	4 (4%)	23 (22%)	12	11 (10%)
Cambria et al. [41]	54	0	16 (30%)	10	2 (4%)	59	1 (2%)	19 (32%)	13	4 (7%)
Butler et al. [43]	32	1 (3%)	8 (25%)	12	2 (6.3%)	15	0	6 (40%)	17	2 (13%)
Rosenbaum et al. [25]*	62	1 (1.6%)	7 (11%)	8	0					
Sicard et al. [42]	70	0	17 (24%)	10	0	75	3 (0.6%)	38 (51%)	13	11 (14%)
Total	876	26 (3%)	201 (23%)	10.5 ± 2.5	11 (1.3%)	531	19 (3.6%)	175 (33%)	15.6 ± 4	44 (8.3%)

*Retroperitoneal approach exclusively under epidural anaesthesia.

concurrent but unrandomized controls [24,25,31,32,39,43]. However, combining all of these analyses gives a total of 1407 patients who underwent aortic surgery via the retroperitoneal ($n = 876$) or transabdominal routes ($n = 531$) (Table 10.2). The operative mortality rate was similar for both groups at 3% and 3.6% for retroperitoneal and transabdominal approaches, respectively, but morbidity in the retroperitoneal group was only 23% compared with 33% for the transperitoneal group. Hospital stay was also reduced in the retroperitoneal group (10.5 ± 2.5 vs 15.6 ± 4 days). Postoperative ileus was seen less often in the retroperitoneal group, occurring in only 1.3% of patients compared with a rate of 8.3% for the transperitoneal group [24,25,30,39,41–43].

Sicard et al., comparing two well-matched but non-randomized groups, observed a significant decrease in postoperative nasogastric intubation (57 vs 98 hours) and an earlier resumption of feeding (3 vs 5 days) in a retroperitoneal versus a transperitoneal group [31]. Similarly, Cambria et al. in their prospective randomized study observed earlier resumption of liquids (3.4 ± 1.3 vs 4.0 ± 1.4 days) and solids (5.1 ± 1.7 vs 6.0 ± 2.2 days) with the retroperitoneal approach [41]. Sicard et al. reported that patients undergoing the retroperitoneal operation had reduced blood loss (1296 ± 109 vs 1950 ± 196 ml (mean $\pm$ s.d.)), required less crystalloids and had better preoperative urinary outputs [31].

Leather et al. also reported a reduced intraoperative blood loss with the retroperitoneal approach (1321 vs 1756 ml) [24]. Butler et al. reported reduced perioperative blood loss using the Risberg retroperitoneal approach (933 ± 586 vs 1100 ± 370 ml) but increased blood loss using a left flank retroperitoneal approach (1300 ± 292 vs 1100 ± 370 ml) compared with transperitoneal controls [43]. However, this group demonstrated a significant decrease ($P > 0.02$) in mean postoperative intubation time (6.5 ± 8 vs 17.3 ± 12 hours), postoperative hospital stay (11 ± 2.4 vs 17.3 ± 7.6 days) and hospital cost (£4885 ± 670 vs £7732 ± 580) with the Risberg retroperitoneal approach compared with the transperitoneal approach [43].

Sicard et al. also estimated the hospitalization costs of the two approaches and calculated that the retroperitoneal approach resulted in a mean saving of US $2587.00 per patient in their series from 1989 (US $12 549 \pm 778$ vs $15 136 \pm 905$ (mean + s.d.)) [31,32]. Finally, Rosenbaum et al. have recently reported a series of 62 patients with aorto-occlusive or aortoiliac disease who underwent infrarenal aortic repair using the retroperitoneal approach where epidural anaesthesia was used exclusively [25]. They demonstrated further reductions in mortality, morbidity and hospital stays compared with historical series performed under general anaesthesia with or without epidural anaesthesia as an adjunct. Interestingly, but not surprisingly, none of the reported complications were of a pulmonary nature [25] (see Table 10.2).

There are a number of theoretical drawbacks to the retroperitoneal approach. Firstly, some time may be spent positioning the patient, but Butler and colleagues, using the Risberg incision, did not find this to be a problem [43]. A frequently quoted disadvantage is the inability to explore the abdomen for other pathology before aneurysm repair. Although associated significant conditions have been reported with abdominal aortic aneurysms, most of these are asymptomatic gallstones [44]. However, preoperative evaluation of patients with abdominal aortic aneurysms using faecal occult blood testing, sonography and computed tomography scanning should detect most unsuspected pathology. Furthermore, the left side of colon, where most colonic malignancies are to be found, is easily palpable through the peritoneum via the retroperitoneal route. Lastly, operating on the aorta via the retroperitoneal approach is technically demanding; access to the right renal artery and/or right iliac system is difficult unless approached from a right-sided flank incision. When access to these vessels is necessary during a left-sided approach, an additional right lower quadrant counterincision is sometimes required.

Physiology of the retroperitoneal approach

Although many authors have observed better results following the retroperitoneal approach for aortic reconstruction [24,30–32,39,42,43], little physiological data exist to explain this benefit. To determine whether the retroperitoneal approach offered any physiological advantage over the transperitoneal approach, Hudson *et al.* [45] compared cardiac dynamics and blood levels of 6-keto-prostaglandin F1α (6-keto-PGF1α) during exposure of the aorta in 56 patients, 33 of whom underwent transabdominal and 19 retroperitoneal exposure of the aorta. They found that mean arterial pressure and systemic vascular resistance decreased and that the cardiac index and heart rate increased and facial flushing occurred 10 minutes after bowel exploration in the transabdominal group. These haemodynamic effects correlated in time and magnitude with a 14-fold increase in 6-keto-PGF1α. None of these changes were observed in patients undergoing retroperitoneal exploration, and these authors speculated that the absence of the response to bowel exploration may account for the observed advantages of the retroperitoneal approach [45].

Further work by Hudson *et al.* [46] has confirmed the hypothesis that prostacyclin is the mediator of the above-mentioned mesenteric traction response and they demonstrated that pretreatment with ibuprofen inhibited these haemodynamic effects during the transperitoneal approach. It, however, remains to be seen whether or not pretreatment agents alone can match the described benefits of the retroperitoneal versus transperitoneal approaches.

In a prospective analysis of 20 patients, O'Sullivan and Bouchier-Hayes [47] compared lung volume and gas exchange changes during and after elective abdominal aortic aneurysm resection using transabdominal ($n = 9$) or retroperitoneal ($n = 11$) routes. They found that intrapulmonary shunting and alveolar/peripheral oxygen gradients were lower in the retroperitoneal group during the cross clamp period and 24 hours after surgery. Functional residual capacity was significantly reduced in the transabdominal group for up to 8 days after the operation. Thus, the retroperitoneal approach was associated with significantly better postoperative oxygenation and preservation of lung volumes. These authors speculated that preservation of diaphragmatic contractility may be better with the retroperitoneal route, and suggested that it may be the preferred approach for elective repair of abdominal aortic aneurysms [47].

Retroperitoneoscopy in vascular surgery

In spite of the explosion of laparoscopy in general surgery in recent years, the application of these techniques to vascular surgery has been almost non-existent. Transthoracic cervicodorsal sympathectomy has long been established and most centres perform this operation thoracoscopically now, the main indication being hyperhydrosis palmaris. The evidence is that the transthoracic approach is easier and safer than the transcervical approach, with the incidence of postoperative Horner's syndrome significantly reduced [48,49].

Retroperitoneoscopy gives an adequate view of the retroperitoneum but this technique has had little application in vascular surgery. One abdominal aortic aneurysm was found coincidentally during retroperitoneal pelvioscopy for staging bladder cancer [50]. However, this is not an ideal method for detecting abdominal aortic aneurysms! Recently, Ahn and colleagues have undertaken laparoscopic aortofemoral bypasses in an experimental pig model with good results. In three of their experiments the approach was retroperitoneal. The proximal anastomosis was achieved using a combination of sutures and titanium clips [51]. Thus, laparoscopic aortic procedures are feasible; whether they are desirable remains to be established. Lumbar sympathectomy is now becoming an infrequent operation in vascular surgery, but theoretically there is no reason why it could not be achieved retroperitoneoscopically with reduced morbidity. However, the main thrust of minimally invasive intervention in vascular surgery remains in the endovascular domain [52].

Conclusion

Since the inauguration of the modern era of aortic surgery by DuBost *et al.* in 1951, a number of surgeons have used the retroperitoneal approach to the infrarenal aorta. The majority of vascular surgeons, however, prefer the transabdominal route. Although the only two prospective randomized trials performed to compare the retroperitoneal and transabdominal approaches to the aorta gave conflicting results [41,42], several retrospective studies attest to the superiority of the retroperitoneal approach. All of the reports document decreased morbidity and hospitalization following this approach [24,29,31,32,39,41,42], all of which are further reduced if the surgery is performed under epidural anaesthesia only [25] (see Table 10.2). The reduced postoperative morbidity associated with retroperitoneal exposure is particularly valuable in the frail, the very old and those with cardiopulmonary disease. Of the various incisions used, Butler and colleagues, comparing two retroperitoneal approaches, found that the lateral paramedian incision carried obliquely onto the chest wall (the Risberg incision) gave the best exposure [43]. While laparoscopic, endoscopic and retroperitoneoscopic approaches to the aorta have been undertaken, maximally invasive surgery remains the standard method for aortic reconstruction. However, we believe that the retroperitoneal route inflicts less biological trauma than the traditional transperitoneal route and suggest that it be considered in all patients undergoing abdominal aortic surgery.

References

1   Jenkins AMcl, Ruckley CV, Nolan B. Ruptured abdominal aortic aneurysms. *Br J Surg* 1986; **73**: 395–8.
2   Thomas PRS, Stewart RD. Abdominal aortic aneurysm. *Br J Surg* 1988; **75**: 733–6.
3   Collin J. Ruptured aortic aneurysms: the coming storm. *Br J Surg* 1987; **74**: 332.
4   Johannsson G, Swedenborg J. Ruptured abdominal aortic aneurysms: a study of incidence and mortality. *Br J Surg* 1986; **73**: 101–3.
5   Ingolby CJH, Wujanto R, Mitchell JE. Impact of vascular surgery on community mortality from ruptured aortic aneurysms. *Br J Surg* 1986; **73**: 551–3.

6 Collin J. Screening for abdominal aortic aneurysms. *Br J Surg* 1985; **72**: 851–2.

7 Crawford ES, Saleh SA, Bubb JW *et al*. Infrarenal abdominal aortic aneurysms. Factors influencing survival after operations performed for a 25 year period. *Ann Surg* 1981; **193**: 699–709.

8 Miturangura P, Stonebridge PA, Clason AE *et al*. Ten year review of non-ruptured aortic aneurysms. *Br J Surg* 1989; **76**: 1251–4.

9 Creech O. Endoaneurysmorrhaphy and treatment of aortic aneurysm. *Ann Surg* 1966; **164**: 935–42.

10 Soreid O, Lillestol J, Christensen O *et al*. Abdominal aortic aneurysms; survival analysis of 434 patients. *Surgery* 1982; **91**: 188–93.

11 Whittlemore AD, Clowes AM, Hechtman HB, Mannick JA. Aortic aneurysm repair: reduced operative mortality associated with maintenance of optimal cardiac performance. *Ann Surg* 1980; **192**: 414–18.

12 Rob C. Extraperitoneal approach to the abdominal aorta. *Surgery* 1963; **53**: 87–9.

13 Sharp WV, Donovan DL. Retroperitoneal approach to the aorta: revisited. *J Cardiovasc Surg* 1987; **28**: 270–3.

14 Abernathy J. *Surgical Observations*. London: Longman & O'Rees, 1804: 209–31.

15 Anon. Dr Murray's case of ligature of the abdominal aorta. *Ann R Coll Surg Engl* 1984; **66**: 408.

16 Cooper A. Case of femoral aneurysm for which the external iliac artery was tied by Sir Astley Cooper Bt: an account of the preparation of the limb, dissected at the expiration of eighteen years. Taken from Sir Astley Cooper's notes. *Guy's Hosp Rep* 1836; **1**: 43–52.

17 Dubost C, Allary M, Oeconomos N. Resection of an aneurysm of the abdominal aorta. *Arch Surg* 1952; **64**: 405–8.

18 Stipa S, Shaw RS. Aorto-iliac reconstruciton through a retroperitoneal approach. *J Cardiovasc Surg* 1968; **9**: 224–36.

19 Helsby R, Moossa AR. Aorto-iliac reconstruction with special reference to the extraperitoneal approach. *Br J Surg* 1975; **62**: 596–600.

20 Stoney RJ, Wylie ET. Surgical management of arterial lesions of the thoracoabdominal aorta. *Am J Surg* 1973; **126**: 157–64.

21 Taheri SA, Gawronski S, Smith D. Paramedian retroperitoneal approach to the abdominal aorta. *J Cardiovasc Surg* 1983; **24**: 529–31.

22 Williams GM, Ricotta JJ, Zinner M, Burdick JD. The extended retroperitoneal approach for the management of extensive atherosclerosis of the aorta and the renal vessels. *Surgery* 1980; **88**: 846–53.

23 Corson JD, Leather RP, Shah DM *et al*. Extraperitoneal aortic bypass with exclusion of the intact infra-renal aortic aneurysm: the *in situ* management of aortic aneurysms. A preliminary report. *J Cardiovasc Surg* 1987; **28**: 274–6.

24 Leather RP, Shah DM, Kaufman JL, Chang BB, Fuestel PJ. Comparative analysis of retroperitoneal and transperitoneal aortic replacement for aneurysm. *Surg Gynecol Obstet* 1989; **168**: 387–93.

25 Rosenbaum GJ, Arroyo PJ, Sivina M. Retroperitoneal approach used exclusively with epidural anaesthesia for intratrenal aortic diesase. *Am J Surg* 1994; **168**: 136–9.

26 Shepard AD, Scott GR, Mackey WC *et al*. Retroperitoneal approach to high risk abdominal aortic aneurysms. *Arch Surg* 1986; **121**: 444–9.

27 Chang BB, Paty PK, Shah DM, Leather RP. Selective use of retroperitoneal aortic exposure in the emergency treatment of ruptured and symptomatic abdominal aortic aneurysms. *Am J Surg* 1988; **156**: 108–10.

28 Shumaker HB Jr. Midline extraperitoneal exposure of the abdominal aorta and iliac arteries. *Surg Gynecol Obstet* 1972; **135**: 791–2.

29 Risberg B, Seeman T, Ortenwall P. A new incision for retroperitoneal approach to the aorta. *Acta Chir Scand* 1989; **155**: 89–91.

30 Metz P, Mathiesen FR. Retroperitoneal approach for implantation of aorto-iliac and aortofemoral vascular prosthesis. *Acta Chir Scand* 1978; **144**: 471–3.

31 Sicard GA, Freeman MB, Vander Woude JC, Anderson CB. Comparison between the transabdominal and retroperitoneal approach for reconstruction of the infrarenal abdominal aorta. *J Vasc Surg* 1987; **5**: 19–27.

32 Sicard GA, Allen BT, Munn JS, Anderson CB. Retroperitoneal versus transperitoneal approach for repair of abdominal aortic aneurysm. *Surg Clin North Am* 1989; **69**: 795–806.

33 Reilly JM, Sicard GA. Right retroperitoneal approaches to the aorta and its branches. *Ann Vasc Surg* 1994; **8**: 318–23.

34 Rosengarten DS, Knight B, Martin P. An approach for operation on the iliac arteries. *Br J Surg* 1971; **58**: 365–6.

35 Bell DD, Gasper M, Movius HJ, Rosenthal JJ, Lemire GG. Retroperitoneal exposure of the terminal aorta and iliac arteries: the Peter Martin approach. *Am J Surg* 1979; **138**: 254–6.

36 Grace PA, Bouchier-Hayes D. Infrarenal abdominal aortic disease: a review of the retroperitoneal approach. *Br J Surg* 1991; **78**: 6–9.

37 Taheri SA, Nowakowski PA, Stoesser FG. Retroperitoneal approach for aortic surgery: experience with 75 consecutive cases. *Vasc Surg* 1969; **69**: 144–8.

38 Darling RC III, Shah DM, Chang BB, Bock DEM, Leather RP. Retroperitoneal approach for bilateral renal and visceral artery revascularization. *Am J Surg* 1994; **168**: 148–51.

39 Johnson JN, McLoughlin GA, Wake PN, Helsby CR, Comparison of extraperitoneal and transperitoneal methods of aortoiliac reconstruction: twenty years experience. *J Cardiovasc Surg* 1986; **27**: 561–4.

40 Mills JL, Fujitani RM, Taylor SM. The retroperitoneal, left flank approach to the supraceliac aorta for difficult and repeat aortic reconstructions. *Am J Surg* 1991; **162**: 638–42.

41 Cambria RP, Brewster DC, Abbott WM *et al*. Transperitoneal versus retroperitoneal approach for aortic reconstruction: a randomized prospective study. *J Vasc Surg* 1990; **11**: 314–25.

42 Sicard GA, Reilly JM, Rubin BG *et al*. Transabdominal versus retroperitoneal incision for abdominal aortic surgery: report of a prospective randomised trial. *J Vasc Surg* 1995; **21**: 174–83.

43 Butler PEM, Grace PA, Broe PJ, Bouchier-Hayes D. Risberg retroperitoneal approach to the abdominal aorta. *Br J Surg* 1993; **80**: 971–3.

44 Thomas JL, McCroskey BL, Iliopoulos JI *et al*. Aortoiliac reconstruction combined with nonvascular operations. *Am J Surg* 1983; **146**: 784–7.

45 Hudson JC, Wurm WH, O'Donnell TF *et al*. Hemodynamic and prostacyclin release in the early phases of aortic surgery: comparison of transabdominal and retroperitoneal approaches. *J Vasc Surg* 1988; **7**: 190–8.

46 Hudson JC, Wurm WH, O'Donnell TF *et al*. Ibuprofen pretreatment inhibits prostacyclin release during abdominal exploration in aortic surgery. *Anesthesiology* 1990; **72**: 443–9.

47 O'Sullivan K, Bouchier-Hayes D. Respiratory function changes: comparison between transabdominal and retroperitoneal approaches for abdominal aortic reconstruction. *Can J Anaesth* 1989; **36**: S71–2.

48 Freidel G, Linder A, Toomes H. Selective video assisted thoracoscopic sympathectomy. *Thorac Cardiovasc Surg* 1993; **41**: 245–8.

49 Ahn SS, Machleder HI, Concepcion B, Moore WS. Thoracoscopic cervicodorsal sympathectomy: preliminary results. *J Vasc Surg* 1994; **20**: 511–17.

50 Ovesen H, Iversen P, Beier-Holgeirsen R *et al*. Extraperitoneal pelviscopy in staging of bladder carcinoma and detection of pelvic lymph node metastasis. *Scand J Urol Nephrol* 1993; **27**: 211–14.

51 Ahn SS, Braithwaite BD, Petrik PV, Clem M. Laparoscopic aortofemoral bypass. *Br J Surg* 1995; **82**: 560.

52 Ahn SS, Eton D, Moore WS. Endovascular surgery for peripheral arterial occlusive disease. A critical review. *Ann Surg* 1992; **216**: 3–16.

Chapter 11

Retroperitoneal laparoscopic aortobifemoral bypass

A.K. Chin and Y-M. Dion

Introduction

Substantial interest currently exists in decreasing the morbidity of aortoiliac revascularization procedures. This interest is illustrated by the efforts of multiple researchers to develop an endovascular technique for repair of abdominal aortic aneurysms [1–4]. Transfemoral placement of stented prosthetic aortic grafts removes the requirement for full length abdominal incisions employed in conventional open aortic repair. Early postprocedural return to normal diet and ambulation may be obtained with endovascular aortic approaches, leading to a decreased hospital stay. Patient recovery is also notable for its lack of pain.

Unfortunately, available endovascular technology is restricted in its application to a select patient population. Transfemoral introduction of a stented graft system is difficult or impossible in patients with small calibre vessels, and in patients with significant infrainguinal atherosclerotic involvement. Iliac tortuosity may also present problems with the endovascular approach, as it inhibits negotiation and placement of the catheter system. Endoluminal graft placement for the treatment of aortic aneurysmal disease requires sufficient infrarenal aortic neck length to allow successful proximal anchoring to occur. Complications also cause concern when endovascular techniques are used in the placement of aortic grafts. Massive microembolization has occurred, and appears to be associated with the presence of substantial intraluminal thrombus in tortuous aortic aneurysms [5]. Stent migration may occur post-treatment, as well as perigraft leakage. The limitations and potential complications experienced with the endovascular approach tempers the enthusiasm surrounding this intriguing technique.

Endoscopic approaches also hold promise for decreasing the magnitude of aortic reconstruction. The ability to provide surgical aortic access without the requirement of full coeliotomy translates directly into decreased surgical morbidity for the patient. Laparoscopically assisted aortobifemoral bypass was first described by Dion *et al.* [6]. Aortic dissection and creation of retroperitoneal tunnels for femoral graft limb passage were performed under a pneumoperitoneal environment, with a total of seven 10 mm trocar ports placed for the introduction of the endoscope, bowel retractors and laparoscopic instruments. The proximal aortic anastomosis was performed in an end-to-side fashion via an 8 cm minilaparotomy incision, following evacuation of gas insufflation. The patient, who had a previous history of three myocardial infarctions, recovered uneventfully and was walking on the second postoperative day.

Laparoscopic aortobifemoral and iliofemoral bypass grafting have also been performed without the use of gas insufflation. Berens and Herde [7] used a transabdominal approach to the aorta, creating an intraperitoneal working space through the use of a mechanical abdominal lift system (Laparolift®, Origin Medsystems, Menlo Park, California, USA) (Fig. 11.1). Their technique involved the initial placement of a lifting fan retractor in the left lower quadrant via a 2 cm incision. Following the addition of instrument ports and a working incision, intra-abdominal laparotomy pads were placed to wall off the bowel. The application of abdominal wall retraction as a substitute for gas insufflation allowed the insertion of conventional open vascular surgical instruments. Bowel retraction, tissue dissection and suture placement were aided by the ability to use non-laparoscopic instrumentation. Potential complications of the pneumoperitoneum, particularly the possibility of gas embolism during the dissection of the great vessels, were also avoided.

Although the ability to successfully perform laparoscopic aortobifemoral bypass is demonstrated by these case examples, present techniques are not suitable for routine application. Significant limitations exist which render the laparoscopic approach cumbersome and difficult to perform. One limitation of current laparoscopic aortic approaches involves the requirement for bowel retraction imposed by transabdominal surgical access. Displacement of the mass of bowel overlying the aorta is generally a formidable task necessitating multiple laparoscopic retractors and various packing schemes. There is always a potential for sudden loss of adequate bowel retraction due to the posterior location of the aorta and the mobility of the large and small bowel covering this structure. Another concern is the ability to obtain adequate vascular control when a limited number of access ports are available for clamp placement. Reliable aortic control must be established, as well as a means of accessing and occluding the lumbar branches. In minimally invasive aortic surgery, complete and immediate access to

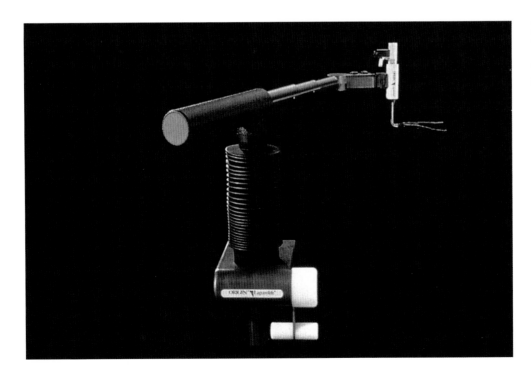

Figure 11.1
The mechanical abdominal lift system used for gasless laparoscopic surgery.

the aorta is unavailable to the surgeon. Instead, the surgeon is removed from the operative site by a distance equal to the depth of the abdominal cavity. A third concern involves the additional operative time required for an endoscopic approach. The increase in operative time is due to several factors. Surgical manipulation requires instrument insertion through trocar ports and multiple instrument exchanges have an additive effect on total procedure length. Limitations in the types and configurations of instruments able to pass through trocar ports or small incisions restrict the dexterity of the surgeon. Simple surgical manoeuvres such as suturing are transformed into cumbersome tasks when using a laparoscopic approach. Delicate and demanding techniques such as those encountered in vascular surgery are magnified in difficulty when a transition to endoscopic surgery is contemplated.

In order to address some of the issues in laparoscopic aortobifemoral bypass surgery, a modified approach and technique is being developed. This technique has been tested in animal and cadaver models, and prelimiary clinical applications are underway.

Surgical technique

The technique involves a gasless total retroperitoneal approach to aortobifemoral reconstruction. Although a standard 10 mm endoscope is applied as in conventional laparoscopy, the technique is atypical as it does not use gas insufflation, the entry incisions and working cavity lie completely outside the peritoneal cavity, and both laparoscopic and open surgical instruments may be inserted into the retroperitoneal space. Essential elements of the technique include the following:

1 Formation of a tract leading to infrarenal retroperitoneal space via a 12 mm flank incision.
2 Dissection of an elongated para-aortic working cavity using an everting balloon cannula.
3 Maintenance of the dissected cavity using a mechanical arm for retraction of the cavity ceiling and an inflatable disc for retraction of the cavity wall.
4 Placement of additional ports and incisions for ancillary instrument access.
5 Isolation of the infrarenal aorta and lumbar arteries at the site of the proximal anastomosis.
6 Aortic crossclamping, aortic transection and performance of the proximal anastomosis.
7 Tunnelling to the groin sites for placement of the femoral anastomoses.
8 Completion of the distal anastomoses.

This technique creates and supports a working laparoscopic cavity extending from the infrarenal aorta down past the aortic bifurcation. The retroperitoneal locale of the cavity makes use of the peritoneum to contain the bowel and intra-abdominal contents, providing a natural plane of retraction. A reliable laparoscopic cavity, essential for aortic manipulation, is achieved.

Formation of an entrance tract

A 15 mm long skin incision is made in the left flank, midway between the lower border of the costal margin and the upper border of the iliac crest, in the anterior-axillary line. The incision is carried down through the subcutaneous layer until the oblique and transversus muscles are identified. Using a pair of curved clamps and the aid of a pair of narrow right-angled retractors, the muscle layers are bluntly separated and retracted to expose the perinephric fatty tissue. The right-angled retractors are removed and an index finger is inserted into the tract to sweep away the loose connective tissue surrounding the lower pole of the kidney. When a plane directly adjacent to the kidney is established, such that the lower border of the kidney may be distinctly palpated, the tract is ready to receive the balloon dissector.

Dissection of the elongated para-aortic cavity

Following the formation of the entrance tract, a specialized balloon cannula (Fig. 11.2) is inserted through this tract into the perinephric space created via finger dissection. The balloon cannula contains an elongated balloon inverted into one lumen of the cannula and accommodates a laparoscope in a separate lumen. Under inflation with a squeeze bulb, the balloon everts from the cannula to dissect an elongated cavity along the course of the aorta, under direct laparoscopic visualization (Fig. 11.3). Following insertion of the cannula into the perinephric space, the cannula is tilted inferiorly to direct the everting balloon along the correct para-aortic plane. The balloon is inflated using regular compressions of the squeeze bulb to perform a controlled dissection along the length of the cavity. A yellowish appearance of the fatty para-aortic tissue will be noted upon endoscopic visualization through the transparent balloon. Full balloon eversion is followed by balloon deflation and removal of the cannula from the entrance tract.

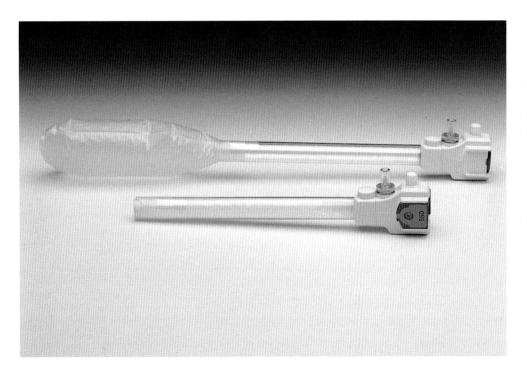

Figure 11.2
The specialized everting balloon cannula used to form an elongated retroperitoneal cavity. The cannula on the top of the photograph shows the fully everted, inflated balloon, while the cannula on the bottom illustrates the initial position of the inverted balloon inside a lumen of the cannula.

Figure 11.3
The placement of the everting balloon cannula in the infrarenal space allows the everting balloon to form an elongated cavity along the course of the aorta.

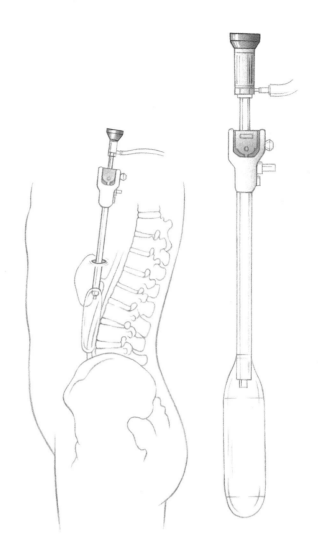

Maintenance of the para-aortic cavity

The dissected retoperitoneal cavity may be supported using a 10 cm length fan retractor (Laparofan®, Origin Medsystems) (Fig. 11.4), elevated by the mechanical lifting arm. The fan retractor is advanced via the insertion tract used for dissection of the elongated cavity and deployed into an open position. Following lifting of the fan retractor, a 12 mm incision is made lateral to the distal end of the outer fan blade to allow insertion of the inflatable balloon retractor for displacement of the medial wall of the cavity (Fig. 11.5). Alternatively, a blunt tip balloon trocar may be used to seal the insertion tract for gas insufflation into the dissected cavity. A retropneumoperitoneum may be used for port placement and the initial stages of aortic dissection, followed by desufflation and conversion of the cavity support to a gasless mechanical technique.

The potential advantage of the preliminary use of gas insufflation in this procedure is the assistance it provides in the placement of ancillary working ports for surgeons unaccustomed to laparoscopy utilizing a gasless technique. Wide lateral expansion of the cavity achieved with gas insufflation simplifies the placement of the first trocar port. With a gasless technique, great care must be taken during insertion of the balloon retractor due to close apposition between

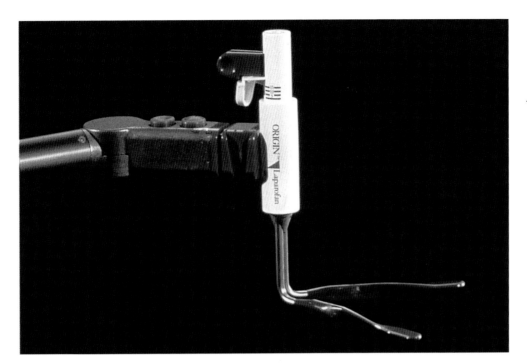

Figure 11.4
The fan retractor used to elevate the ceiling of the retroperitoneal cavity. The fan retractor is lifted by the powered mechanical arm.

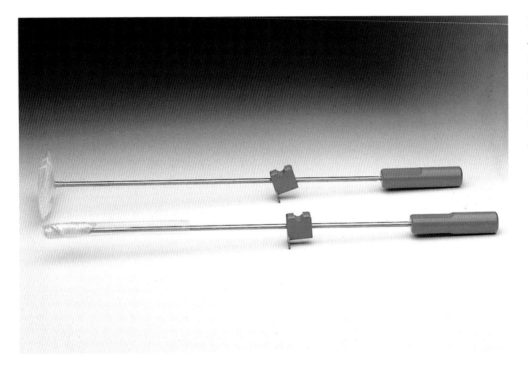

Figure 11.5
A version of the balloon retractor used to displace the medial wall of the retroperitoneal cavity. The retractor is shown in its uninflated and inflated states.

the medial and lateral walls of the retroperitoneal cavity prior to the establishment of medial retraction. Once the medial balloon retractor is placed, however, ample space exists for the insertion of additional ports or instruments. As additional experience is gained with gasless techniques in laparoscopic surgery, the surgeon may forego the step of initial gas insufflation and proceed directly to mechanical cavity retraction, saving both time and inconvenience associated with carbon dioxide instillation.

Working port placement

Three additional incisions are placed for instrument access in retroperitoneal laparoscopic aortic reconstruction. Two lateral sites are added superior to the balloon retractor insertion site. One incision is performed midway along the blade of the fan retractor and the other lateral incision is placed at the level of the original dissection tract now occupied by the fan retractor. Both incisions are placed approximately 3 cm lateral to the border of the outer lifting fan blade. The last incision is placed several centimetres superior to the dissection tract incision; this incision is used for proximal aortic cross clamp placement. With gasless laparoscopy, simple stab incisions may be used to provide sites for instrument access. Each incision site may accommodate two or more 5 mm diameter laparoscopic instruments. If frequent instrument exchanges through a particular incision are contemplated, a simple valveless flexible port is inserted to reserve a pathway through the peritoneum for unrestricted instrument passage. Additionally, if the flexible port is slit lengthwise along one plane, conventional open surgical instruments with hinged pivot points may be opened as if the port were not present within the incision. Maximal flexibility is achieved while maintaining access through the entire length of the incision.

Aortic dissection

The elongated cavity formed by balloon dissection greatly facilitates the task of aortic dissection (Fig. 11.6). Isolation of the infrarenal aorta is performed with several centimetres of the aorta dissected free in a circumferential manner. Laparoscopic dissection instruments may be used for this exposure, as well as a long pair of right-angle clamps. Following dissection, a loop of silastic or umbilical tape is placed encircling the aorta. Lumbar vessels observed in the vicinity of the exposed infrarenal aortic segment are ligated or clipped using titanium clips. Distally, a second segment of the aorta is isolated and a vessel loop placed to allow control of back bleeding upon transection of the aorta and subsequent graft placement.

Figure 11.6
Appearance of the retroperitoneal cavity maintained in a gasless state using the mechanical lift and balloon retraction.

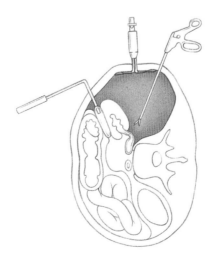
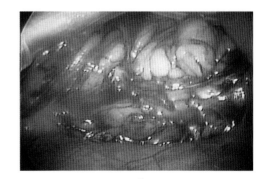

Aortic graft placement

The aortic cross clamp is inserted just below the renal arteries, distal to the proximal vessel loop previously placed. The proximal vessel loop is maintained for added security in this situation of limited aortic accessibility imposed by the laparoscopic approach. The aorta is transected approximately 2 cm distal to the cross clamp, using a pair of Potts' scissors or laparoscopic shears. The prosthetic graft is advanced into the retroperitoneal cavity via one of the lateral access incisions, and a grasper is used to position the proximal end of the graft adjacent to the transected end of the aorta. The posterior wall is sutured first using a continuous stitch within the lumen of the vessel (Fig. 11.7). The intraluminal running suture is preceded by a knot, and upon completion of the posterior wall anastomosis, the free end of the suture is left long. The anterior wall is then sewn with a separate strand of suture using an extraluminal technique. Following this, the free end of the anterior suture is tied to the free end of the posterior suture, completing the proximal end-to-end anastomosis.

Groin site tunnel formation

Bilateral groin incisions are performed to isolate the common, superficial and deep femoral arteries on both sides, and vessel loops are placed on the respective branches. Access tunnels are formed in a retrograde manner, from the groin incisions back towards the retroperitoneal space. Vascular graft tunnellers with a distal tapered conical tip and an outer sleeve are passed along the course of the common femoral and external iliac arteries, under the inguinal ligament and into the elongated laparoscopic cavity. Passage of the tunneller into the retroperitoneal cavity may be conducted under endoscopic guidance to ensure an atraumatic entry in the proper location. Use of the fan retractor and mechanical

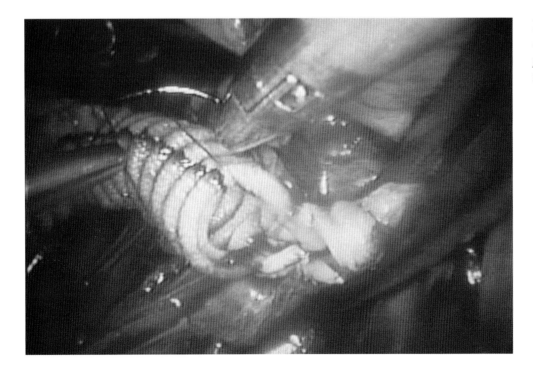

Figure 11.7
Suture placement in the posterior wall of the transected aorta.

arm as a cavity support is helpful during the tunnelling process. Entrance into the retroperitoneal space is not associated with a loss of visualization, as is experienced with gas insufflation. Following tunnel formation, laparoscopic graspers may be threaded into the retroperitoneal cavity to retrieve the femoral limb of the prosthetic graft on either side. Care is taken to prevent twisting or kinking of the graft during this process.

Distal anastomosis

The retrieved limbs of the bifurcated aortic graft are anastomosed to the common femoral artery in an end-to-side fashion in the customary manner. After a final check has been performed to make sure that haemostasis has been achieved at both the proximal and distal anastomotic sites, the various incisions are closed. Instrument access sites in the retroperitoneum are closed with the fan retractor in an elevated position which allows incisional closure under laparoscopic vision. The fan insertion site is closed last.

Experimental results

A porcine model was used to evaluate the retroperitoneal laparoscopic approach to the aorta. Nineteen pigs, with weights ranging from 60 to 78 kg, underwent aortic dissection via a retroperitoneal approach with the laparoscopic cavity prepared by balloon dissection. The cavity was examined under gas insufflation and isolation of the infrarenal aorta was initiated under a retropneumoperitoneum. Gas insufflation was replaced with mechanical retraction, using the powered lifting arm, to permit aortic dissection to be completed under a gasless laparoscopic environment. Isolation of the aorta extended from the origin of the left artery down past the aortic bifurcation. Lumbar arteries encountered during the dissection were ligated with laparoscopic titanium clips.

In four animals, aortobifemoral bypass was completed using a bifurcated graft. The proximal anastomosis was performed in an end-to-end fashion using a running suture of 4/0 Prolene. The distal anstomoses were completed with 5/0 Prolene, in an end-to-side manner with the common femoral artery, bilaterally. Formation of a tract between the groin incisions and the retroperitoneal space was carried out with a curved tunnelling device (Laborie Surgical, Canada). Anticoagulation during the procedures was accomplished with systemic heparinization, with an initial dose of 100 IU/kg followed 90 minutes later by an additional dose of 50 IU/kg if the anastomoses were still in process.

All aortobifemoral procedures were completed in less than 4 hours; the last procedure required a total operative time of 3 hours. All procedures were completed successfully. Blood loss did not exceed 250 cm^3, and most of the blood loss occurred during the release of the proximal aortic cross clamp. Proximal anastomotic leakage was present in two of the cases. In one case, the leak was limited to a slight oozing which was controlled with the application of a collagen sponge. In the other case, two interrupted sutures were placed to stop the leakage.

Discussion

A retroperitoneal approach to laparoscopic aortic surgery addresses the issue of aortic access in the presence or overlying bowel. Limitations of a transabdominal laparoscopic approach to the aorta have been recognized by many clinicians involved in the development of endoscopic aortic reconstruction techniques. The requirement for bowel control is one reason for the degree of technical difficulty associated with laparoscopic aortobifemoral bypass procedures. The mobility and sheer volume of bowel tends to overwhelm the capacity of single or even multiple laparoscopic retractors to contain the bowel and provide proper aortic exposure. The substantial increase in procedure length of laparoscopic versus open aortic surgery reflects the additional demands imposed by a transabdominal endoscopic approach. The advantage that a peritoneum confers, as an envelope which contains the entire mass of bowel and segregates it from the operative aortic field, cannot be overemphasized. With the establishment of a retroperitoneal operating cavity, the kidney remains as the only structure that requires retraction. All other instruments may direct their attention to the isolation and manipulation of the aorta.

The combined use of gasless laparoscopy and total retroperitoneal aortic access serves to enhance vascular control in the face of limited instrument entry sites. Mechanical retraction with the fan and powered lifting arm provides positive support of the para-aortic operating cavity. The potential loss of surgical exposure due to the escape of gas insufflation is not a concern. If desirable or necessary, digital palpation of the aorta is available. The mechanical lifting arm may be lowered to bring the ceiling of the endoscopic cavity closer to the aorta, and an index finger may be inserted through an access incision to evaluate the aorta for presence of calcification and to identify the proper anastomotic location. A gasless environment enables conventional vascular needle holders and clamps to be inserted into the retroperitoneal cavity. Mini incisions accommodate the use of open surgical instruments, reducing the awkwardness often associated with long-shafted laparoscopic instruments. Generally, a mixture of laparoscopic and non-laparoscopic instruments are applied during gasless retroperitoneal aortic surgery. In some situations it may be preferable to use a laparoscopic instrument, with its small profile and extended length; for example, during dissection of the aortic bifucation via a proximal instrument port. In other situations the ability to use conventional open instruments increases the ease of surgical manipulation; for example, the application of a right-angled clamp to place a vessel loop around the aorta.

Maintenance of the retroperitoneal cavity using a mechanical lift system benefits the aortobifemoral procedure in additional ways. Continuous suction aspiration may be utilized during electrocautery use. In the event of significant bleeding, high flow suction may be applied without incurring working cavity loss due to desufflation. Femoral access may be accomplished under endoscopic control without visual interruption upon the entrance of the tunnelling device into the retroperitoneal space. A gasless approach also alleviates concerns regarding complications associated with carbon dioxide insufflation. Acidosis due to high carbon dioxide absorption rates in the dissected retroperitoneal space and gas embolism resulting from vascular entry in a pressurized gaseous environment are potential complications removed by the use of the mechanical lift system.

The total retroperitoneal gasless laparoscopic approach to aortobifemoral bypass circumvents some of the issues experienced with endovascular aortic reconstruction. Successful graft placement is not limited by small native vessel size or iliac tortuosity. Negotiation through a thrombus-laden aorta is not required with a laparoscopic technique, reducing concern over the potential occurrence of a massive microembolization. A standard end-to-end suture anastomosis is performed removing the incidence of stent migration. The endoscopic approach seeks to preserve important technical aspects of open aortic bypass surgery and to accomplish these techniques in a closed cavity enviroment. With this approach, the advantages of traditional open vascular reconstruction are combined with the benefits of minimal incision surgery.

Conclusion

The development of additional techniques and instrumentation is needed to allow laparoscopic aortobifemoral bypass surgery to become a practical, widespread procedure. The balloon-assisted, gasless retroperitoneal approach outlined in this chapter addresses the issues of aortic access and surgical retraction critical to the success of any endoscopic aortic reconstructive endeavour. Continued research along these lines will hopefully make this endeavour a reality.

References

1   Parodi JC, Palmaz JC, Barone HD. Transfemoral intraluminal graft implantation for abdominal aortic aneurysms. *Ann Vasc Surg* 1991; **5**: 491–9.

2   Volodos NL, Karpovich IP, Troyan VI *et al*. Clinical experience of the use of self-fixing synthetic prosthesis for remote endoprosthetics of the thoracic and the abdominal aorta and iliac arteries through the fermoral artery and as intraoperative endoprosthesis for aorta reconstruction. *Vasa Suppl* 1991; **33**: 93–5.

3   Chuter TAM, Green RM, Ouriel K *et al*. Transfemoral endovascular aortic graft placement. *J Vasc Surg* 1993; **18**: 185–97.

4   Marin ML, Veith FJ, Cynamon J *et al*. Transfemoral endovascular stented graft treatment of aortoiliac and femoropopliteal occlusive disease for limb salvage. *Am J Surg* 1994; **168**: 156–62.

5   Parodi JC. Endovascular repair of abdominal aortic aneurysms and other arterial lesions. In: Szabo Z, Kerstein MD, Lewis JE, eds. *Surgical Technology International III*. San Franciso: Universal Medical Press, 1994: 431–6.

6   Dion YM, Katkhouda N, Rouleau C *et al*. Laparoscopy-assisted aortobifemoral bypass. *Surg Laparosc Endosc* 1993; **3**(5): 425–9.

7   Berens E, Herde J. Laparoscopic aortobifemoral bypass. Presented to the Vascular Surgery Motion Picture Session of the 70th Clinical Congress of the American College of Surgeons, October 1994.

Chapter 12

Balloon-assisted extraperitoneal surgery

A.K. Chin and F.H. Moll

Introduction

The ability of laparoscopic surgery to reduce the extent of operative incisions and subsequent postoperative morbidity is well recognized. Successful application of a laparoscopic technique to intraperitoneal procedures such as cholecystectomy, appendectomy and vaginal hysterectomy makes its extension to other open surgical procedures desirable. In order to perform endoscopic surgery, achievement of two technical functions is required. The first function is the formation and maintenance of a surgical working cavity. The second requirement is the acquisition and display of visual images, via rigid or fibreoptic telescopes with video camera transmission to a video monitor. Once an operating cavity with visualization capability is established, laparoscopic surgical instruments may be introduced to perform the minimally invasive procedure.

Creation of an intra-abdominal cavity for laparoscopic surgery is a routine procedure, with carbon dioxide (CO_2) gas insufflation employed to form a pneumoperitoneum. Mechanical means of lifting the abdominal wall are also described [1–3]; these methods may offer a substitute for gas insufflation and the potential for conventional surgical instrument use in laparoscopy.

Laparoscopy affords access to abdominal organs; however, a significant number of vital structures lie in the extraperitoneal space, either in the retroperitoneum or in the preperitoneum. Endoscopic techniques may be applied to extraperitoneal structures, yielding similar clinical benefits to those observed in laparoscopic surgery. Although extraperitoneal organs are accessible via transabdominal laparoscopic approaches, these techniques are cumbersome, requiring entry into the belly followed by exit from the peritoneal cavity to reach the target organ. Passage through the abdominal cavity complicates the procedure by adding a requirement for bowel retraction. Multiple instruments are inserted for the sole purpose of bowel displacement. The bowel must be cleared from the surgical site for initial access and for the duration of the procedure. A transabdominal approach to extraperitoneal endoscopic surgery also exposes the patient to increased risk of postoperative abdominal adhesion formation and potential bowel herniation through unapproximated edges of incised peritoneum.

Direct access to the extraperitoneal endoscopic operative site is desired to avoid the limitations encountered with an indirect, transabdominal approach. The retroperitoneal or preperitoneal cavity created for operative use is formed in a potential space composed of soft connective tissue. This is in contrast to conventional laparoscopy, which occurs in the predetermined space of the abdominal cavity with natural demarcations delineated by the peritoneal boundary.

Previous authors have described techniques for retroperitoneal endoscopic surgery. In 1976, Wittmoser [4] outlined his technique for retroperitoneoscopy as an approach to lumbar sympathectomy.

Blunt dissection with the tip of the endoscope is accompanied by CO_2 insufflation in the retroperitoneal space to create a large working cavity for sympathectomy or lymphadenectomy. Other surgeons have applied a combination of mechanical dissection and gas insufflation to the preperitoneal space for laparoscopic inguinal hernia repair and lymph node dissection. Ferzli *et al.* [5] describe the use of a 10 mm working endoscope with a blunt probe advanced through the 5 mm working channel to dissect the preperitoneal cavity, which is maintained with CO_2 insufflation, to accomplish staging pelvic lymphadenectomy. McKernan and Laws [6] employed a similar approach to prepare a preperitoneal endoscopic cavity for inguinal herniorrhaphy.

The blunt dissection techniques described above result in extraperitoneal cavities with roughly dissected internal surfaces, Strands of extraperitoneal connective tissue and fat crisscross the manually dissected space, making it difficult to identify anatomical landmarks. Difficulties with blunt dissections and subsequent surgical visualization limit the widespread use of these techniques and reserve their application to surgeons with significant laparoscopic experience.

The search for simple, reliable methods of tissue separation in the extraperitoneal space led to the development of balloon devices for blunt dissection. Balloon inflation is a practical means of cavity formation in loose connective tissue layers. Its application enables the surgeon to create a predictable working environment in the desired extraperitoneal location. The resultant cavity contains a smooth surface, and minimal bleeding is noted post-dissection.

History of balloon-assisted extraperitoneal surgery

Gaur [7] published a report in 1992 concerning the balloon preparation of an endoscopic retroperitoneal surgical cavity, using a surgical glove tied to a red rubber catheter and inflated with a pneumatic squeeze bulb. The fingers of the surgical glove were suture ligated and amputated, and the cavity was maintained using gas insufflation at pressures between 5 and 10 mmHg. Retroperitoneal laparoscopic procedures performed with this technique included ureterolithotomy, renal biopsy, para-aortic lymph node biopsy and internal spermatic vein ligation. Other researchers reported similar techniques of balloon dilatation in the retroperitoneal and preperitoneal spaces. Keizur *et al.* [8] applied a combination of Foley balloon catheter inflation followed by surgical glove dilatation to perform retroperitoneal laparoscopic renal biopsies. Kieturakis [9] describes a relatively inelastic balloon cannula inflated with saline in the preperitoneal space as a technique for preparing a working space for laparoscopic hernia repair.

The forementioned cavity dissection techniques employ the blind application of the dilating medium in the extraperitoneal space. A cannula (Fig. 12.1) combining balloon dilatation and direct visualization of the dissection process was described by Chin *et al.* [10] in 1994. The cannula shaft accommodates a

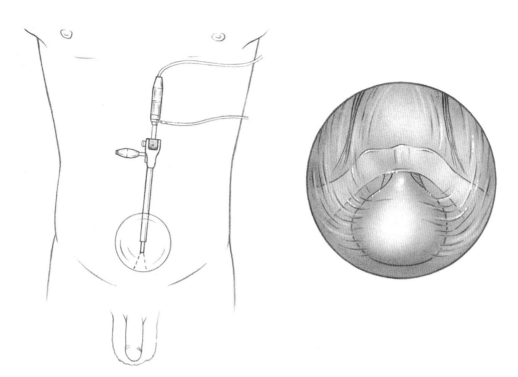

Figure 12.1
The direct visualization balloon dissection cannula.

laparoscope, the distal trip of which lies within the balloon to permit evaluation of the initial cannula placement, the dissection progress and the final cavity size. Balloon inflation with the pneumatic squeeze bulb is continued until an adequate working space is appreciated upon endoscopic inspection. This dissection technique has been used for laparoscopic inguinal herniorrhaphy, pelvic lymphadenectomy [11], varicocele ligation, nephropexy, renal biopsy, implantation of the inguinal reservoir of inflatable penile prostheses [12] and bladder neck suspension. Direct visualization balloon dilators have been developed with both elastic and relatively inelastic balloons. The elastic balloons form a spherical cavity suitable for centrally located procedures such as bladder neck suspension, while the inelastic balloons dissect out alternate configurations and permit lateral extension of the preperitoneal cavity required during bilateral hernia repair procedures.

Mechanical considerations

Visual balloon dissection of the extraperitoneal space is performed with a simple cannula consisting of a single-chambered balloon and a conventional laparoscope. Following extraperitoneal cavity formation, a separate cannula with a small distal balloon is used to seal the entrance tract leading to the dissected space, and CO_2 insufflation is introduced to maintain the working environment. Technical considerations relevant to a laparoscopic extraperitoneal surgical approach include the choice of dissection balloon material, the configuration of the dissection cannula and the method used to support the surgical cavity.

Dissection balloon material

Two categories of balloon material are used for extraperitoneal dissection; these include an elastomeric material and a generally inelastic plastic material.

An elastic balloon inflates to a spherical shape, and the elasticity of the material allows the balloon to assume a small deflated profile. Visualization is achieved at the outset of cannula placement, prior to balloon inflation. Following advancement of the elastic balloon in the extraperitoneal plane, the laparoscope is inserted into the cannula and the tissue outside the balloon may be appreciated through the transparent balloon material. Correct positioning of the balloon is verified by noting the yellowish appearance of the extraperitoneal fatty tissue, before proceeding with balloon inflation. Improper cannula insertion into a superficial muscle plane is denoted by a pink visual field outside of the balloon, while inadvertant passage through the peritoneum is characterized by the appearance of bowel viewed through the laparoscope. Early viewing through the dissection cannula avoids large peritoneal tears caused by balloon inflation with the cannula in an incorrect position.

During inflation of an elastomeric dissection balloon, back pressure is experienced through the pneumatic squeeze bulb. The majority of the pressure in the balloon is exerted on the wall of the balloon, causing it to expand. The remainder of the pressure serves to dissect the extraperitoneal cavity. This situation is in contrast to inelastic balloons, in which internal inflation pressure in the oversized balloon correlates more closely with the force exerted directly on tissue during dissection. An elastomeric dissection balloon is capable of dissecting a range of cavity sizes, while an inelastic balloon is limited to a specific maximal volume.

Inelastic material is chosen when the balloon is used to form specific cavity shapes. An inelastic balloon inflates to a given size and shape, and increased inflation pressure does not enlarge the dissected cavity dimensions. The inelastic balloon is rolled about the axis of the cannula for initial placement. Endoscopic placement within the balloon is not performed until early partial balloon inflation has formed a small internal balloon channel to accommodate the laparoscope. Inelastic balloons may be formed with varied configurations so desired cavity aspect ratios of height, width and depth can be achieved.

Functional concerns regarding balloon dissection in the extraperitoneal space include overdistension and the potential for air embolism upon balloon rupture. Direct endoscopic visualization during balloon inflation allays fear of injury during tissue dissection, as the scope monitors the progress of dissection to the desired endpoint in cavity size. Also, the dissection capacity in the extraperitoneal space is voluminous. J. Himpens (personal communication) reports that dissection volumes of 5 litres may be routinely achieved in patients undergoing retroperitoneoscopy. The potential for air embolism upon balloon rupture is practically non-existent, due to the presence of open communication between the dissected cavity and the outside of the patient, and the low balloon inflation pressure used during extraperitoneal dissection. The entrance tract made to permit the introduction of the balloon cannula is sufficiently large to accommodate the balloon end of the dissection cannula. The distal end of the cannula, which bears the balloon, has a larger diameter than the proximal cannula shaft, ensuring that clearance space exists between the cannula and the surrounding tissue tract for immediate equalization of internal and external pressure in the event of balloon rupture.

Balloon cannula configuration

The elastomeric balloon dissection cannula (Fig. 12.2) has a balloon at the end of the cannula with an inner tube that extends to the distal tip of the deflated balloon, providing axial balloon support during insertion and advancement. An obturator fits into the cannula, filling the open end of the cannula with a smooth, rounded tip. The proximal end of the cannula houses a valve, which seals against the 10 mm laparoscope inserted into the balloon following obturator removal. The valve contains a button-controlled flap door that opens to deflate the balloon following cavity dissection. An inflation port accepts the pneumatic bulb used to inject air into the balloon.

The inelastic balloon dissection cannula contains an identical-sized cannula and valve housing. However, the inner cannula consists of a thin metal tube that extends to the distal end of the balloon, which is rolled about the tube and covered with a plastic sheath for smooth introduction. The sheath is longitudinally perforated, splitting open upon balloon inflation. Following initial balloon inflation, the laparoscope is inserted into the balloon to monitor the remainder of the dissection.

Cavity support

Upon completion of the extraperitoneal balloon dissection, the balloon cannula is deflated and removed from the body. A blunt tip trocar port with a small distal balloon is inserted into the dissection tract, forming a gastight seal for CO_2 insufflation (Fig. 12.3). The port compresses the incision between an internally placed toroidal balloon and an external foam cuff which clamps against the skin surface. Additional instrument ports may be inserted under direct visual guidance, using a laparoscope placed through the blunt tip trocar.

The balloon-dissected extraperitoneal cavity may also be maintained without the use of gas insufflation. A mechanical lift system (Laparolift, Origin Medsystems, Menlo Park, California, USA) may be inserted through the dissection balloon tract and used to support the ceiling of the surgical cavity. This system uses a fan retractor which is inserted through the dissection tract and deployed to form a triangular plane of lift for the surgical cavity (Fig.12.4). An additional mechanical or inflatable retractor is advanced into the cavity via a

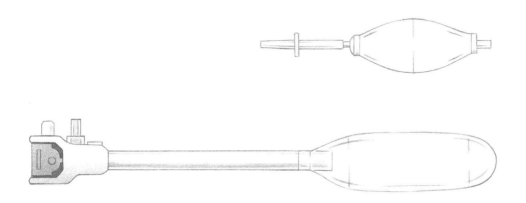

Figure 12.2
The components of the elastomeric balloon dissection cannula.

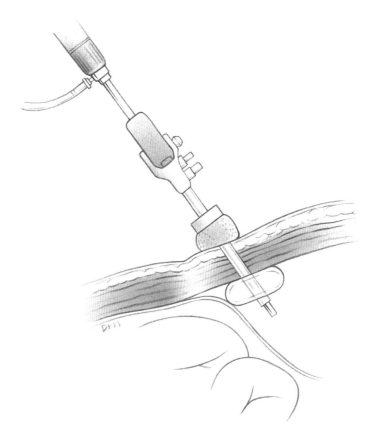

separate incision, to support the medial wall of the surgical space. Non-insufflation means of supporting the extraperitoneal cavity contribute benefits in terms of technical approach and surgical instrument application. Conventional open surgical instruments may be applied through small skin incisions, without the requirement for laparoscopic trocar sleeves. Endoscopic suturing and tissue manipulation may be simplified by returning to traditional instrumentation, with the potential for improved surgical control and decreased operative time.

Surgical technique

Balloon-assisted extraperitoneal dissection is a simple technique involving skin incision, blunt dissection to the level of the preperitoneum, initiation of the insertion tract via finger dissection, advancement and inflation of the balloon cannula under direct vision and maintenance of the working cavity via the blunt-tipped insufflation cannula or the mechanical lifting retractor.

Preperitoneal cavity formation

Access to the preperitoneal plane may be performed via an infaumbilical midline incision, carried down through the linea alba. With this approach, however, it is relatively easy to inadvertently enter the peritoneum — either upon the initial incision or during the introduction of the balloon cannula. A more reliable technique of balloon cannula insertion involves an off-midline dissection through the rectus muscle (Fig. 12.5). If a midline skin incision is preferred for cosmetic reasons, the incision is retracted laterally to enter the rectus sheath. A 12 mm

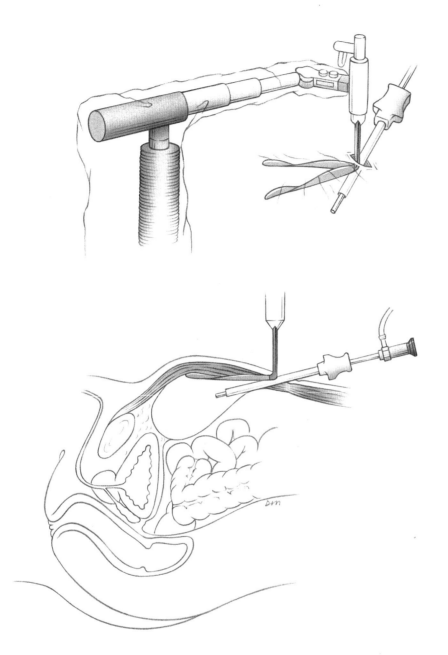

Figure 12.4
*The mechanical lift system
and fan retractor.*

incision is made in the anterior rectus sheath. The underlying rectus muscle is retracted to expose the posterior rectus sheath. An index finger is used to initiate a tract between the rectus muscle and the posterior rectus sheath, and the balloon cannula is advanced inferiorly through this tract. If a midline preperitoneal cavity is desired, for laparoscopic bladder neck suspension or lymphadenectomy procedures, the balloon cannula is directed towards the pubic symphysis. A gentle twisting motion is applied to the cannula during advancement. The axis of the cannula is maintained in a plane parallel to the abdominal wall; this prevents the cannula from entering the rectus muscle or puncturing through the peritoneum into the abdominal cavity. The tip of the cannula may be palpated through the skin to verify its final position.

Following dissection cannula placement, the obturator is removed, and a laparoscope advanced into the cannula 1 cm short of the distal tip. Appreciation

Figure 12.5
Preperitoneal cavity formation via a paramedian incision. The steps of balloon dissection and blunt tip trocar placement are shown.

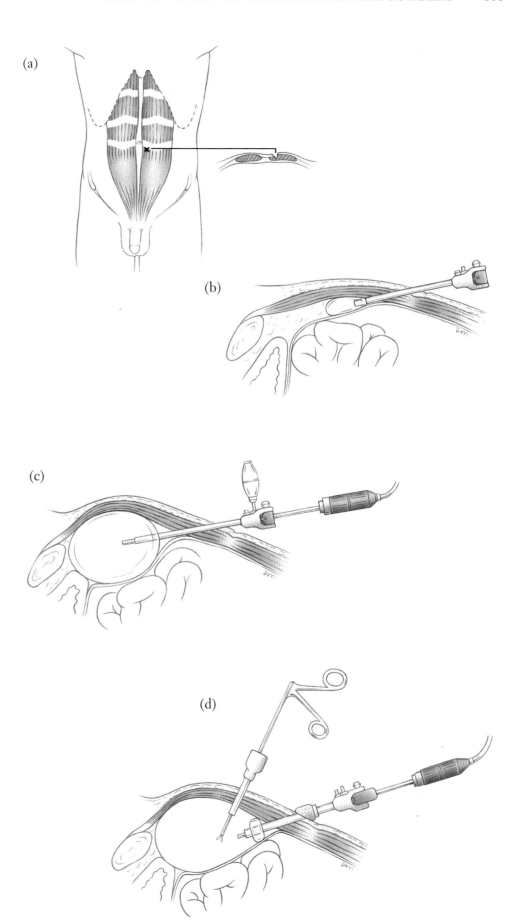

of yellow coloration indicative of preperitoneal fat assures the surgeon of correct placement, and balloon inflation is performed. The laparoscope is advanced into the centre of the balloon and it may be pivoted in all directions to visualize the landmarks within the cavity. Balloon dissection is continued until a sufficient working space is achieved, or to a maximal volume of approximately 1 litre.

Retroperitoneal cavity formation

An access incision for the balloon cannula is performed in the mid- to posterior axillary line, midway between the costal margin and the iliac crest (Fig. 12.6). The 12–15 mm incision is carried down to the external and internal oblique muscles, which are spread apart using a pair of curved clamps to reach the perinephric region. Blunt finger dissection is conducted to displace the areolar fatty tissue surrounding the kidney, until its lower pole is palpated. The balloon cannula is advanced through this tract, the laparoscope inserted into the cannula, and the balloon inflated to form an infrarenal cavity. Following deflation and removal of the dissection balloon cannula, the blunt tip balloon trocar is placed in the dissection tract and gas insufflation initiated to maintain the cavity. Additional trocar ports are inserted into the retroperitoneal space under direct visualization by the laparoscope, which is introduced through the blunt tip balloon trocar.

The spherical elastomeric balloon cannula is generally used for retroperitoneal dissection during laparoscopic nephrectomy or adrenalectomy procedures. For aortic procedures, a specialized inelastic balloon cannula is applied (see Chapter 9). This cannula dissects an elongated cavity along the abdominal aorta, from the infrarenal area to the aortic bifurcation. If an expanded proximal cavity is desired, the elastomeric balloon cannula may be inserted following dissection of the elongated portion.

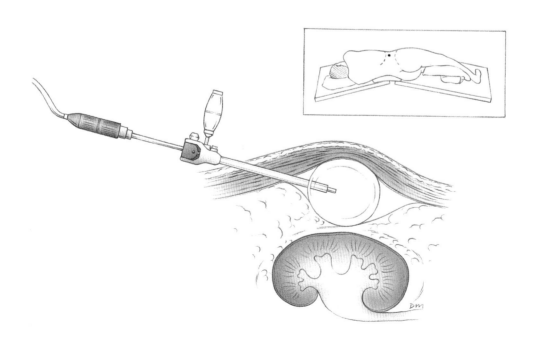

Figure 12.6
The access site for retroperitoneal balloon dissection.

Clinical applications

Inguinal hernia repair

Total preperitoneal hernia repair provides benefits in terms of avoiding peritoneal violation and offering the potential for herniorrhaphy under regional or local anaesthesia. Balloon preparation of the preperitoneal space results in an improved appearance of the surgical cavity, with an enhanced delineation of the anatomical landmarks. The preperitoneal space is characterized by the presence of a significant amount of fatty tissue, which makes it difficult to appreciate normal hernia landmarks visible from a transabdominal approach. With balloon dissection, the white arch of Cooper's ligament takes a prominent appearance and the remaining landmarks can be identified in relation to this ligament. Proceeding laterally from the pubic symphysis, the iliac vessels are noted to cross Cooper's ligament. The epigastric vessels originate from the iliac vessels and course upwards in the preperitoneal cavity, towards the internal inguinal ring. If a unilateral hernia repair is conducted, a spherical elastomeric balloon cannula may be used for the dissection with the balloon directed towards the involved side via a periumbilical incision. If bilateral herniorrhaphy is performed, an inelastic balloon with an elliptical configuration is applied to dissect a preperitoneal cavity that extends adequately to both sides for a proper mesh repair.

Burch procedure

Midline placement of the elastomeric balloon dissection cannula is used to prepare a working cavity encompassing the vesicourethral junction. Blunt dissection is performed to delineate the proximal urethra, and one or more suture strands are placed between the periurethral tissue and Cooper's ligament above and lateral to the urethra. The 1 litre cavity size is adequate to permit placement of bilateral periurethral suspension sutures. Knots tied in an extracorporeal fashion are cinched down with a knot pusher to produce the desired tension. Equal suture tension is applied bilaterally to achieve a symmetrical suspension of the bladder neck.

Additional preperitoneal procedures

Additional laparoscopic procedures that may be performed using a total preperitoneal approach include pelvic lymphadenectomy and implantation of the prevesical reservoir of an inflatable penile prosthesis. Total preperitoneal pelvic lymph node dissection allows minimally invasive surgical staging of patients with carcinoma of the prostate. Preperitoneal endoscopic cavity formation is performed using the elastomeric dissection balloon cannula, which is advanced in the midline inferiorly from an infraumbilical incision to provide access to the iliac vessels bilaterally. Dissection of the lymphatic chain is carried out along the course of the external iliac vein, from the iliac bifurcation distally to the circumflex iliac vein [13].

The multicomponent inflatable penile prosthesis requires a 100 cm^3 inguinal reservoir to be placed in the prevesical space; this space may be formed by inflation of the elastomeric balloon cannula [12]. Inflation of the dissection cannula with 200 cm^3 of air creates the cavity with a decreased potential for bladder injury which may occur with conventional mechanical blunt dissection.

Retroperitoneal procedures

Formation of a retroperitoneal endoscopic cavity affords access to the kidney, the adrenal gland, the ureter, the aorta and the lumbar spine. Initial access for the placement of the dissection balloon cannula is accomplished via a 2 cm flank incision, approximately 2 cm above the iliac crest in the mid-axillary line [11]. Blunt finger dissection is carried out to form a tract through the muscular planes, until the perinephric region is reached. The dissection balloon is advanced into the fibrous septa occupying the retroperitoneal area. The cannula is directed superiorly to create a cavity for nephrectomy, adrenalectomy or nephropexy. An inferior orientation of the cannula is used for access to the spermatic vessels, the aorta and the lower spine. Aortic isolation is accomplished using a specialized everting inelastic balloon cannula, as described in Chapter 11.

Keizur *et al.* [8] describe a technique for retroperitoneal laparoscopic renal biopsy, using blind dissection with a 22F Foley balloon catheter, followed by saline inflation of a surgical glove with knotted fingers in the same space. Exposure of the lower pole of the kidney is performed using blunt dissection under gas insufflation in the retroperitoneal cavity. Continued dissection in the same cavity may be used for nephrectomy and adrenalectomy. Retraction of the kidney exposes the renal hilum for isolation of the renal vessels. Rassweiler *et al.* [14] incised the ureter and used it as a tether to assist with kidney retraction during transperitoneal laparoscopic nephrectomy. A similar technique may be applied during total retroperitoneal laparoscopic nephrectomy. Occlusion and transection of the renal artery and vein may be performed using suture ligation or through the use of endoscopic stapling devices.

Experimental lumbar discectomy has been performed using a gasless retroperitoneal laparoscopic approach. Balloon dissection of an inferiorly directed retroperitoneal cavity is accomplished via a flank incision, as described above, and maintained through the use of a Laparolift and an additional balloon retractor for displacement of the peritoneum along the medial aspect of the cavity. The aorta and vena cava are partially isolated and retracted medially; the psoas muscle is dissected and retracted laterally to expose the anterior portion of the spine. Dissectomy is performed using conventional periosteal elevators and laminectomy rongeurs.

Future developments

Various concepts are presently under development in order to improve the technical aspects of balloon dissection and extraperitoneal cavity maintenance. New balloon dissection concepts include methods to obtain increased dissection in the transverse plane, asymmetrical dissection and methods to combine the functions of cavity formation and cavity maintenance into a single device. Additional research is being conducted to improve retraction capabilities within the extraperitoneal endoscopic space.

Dissection of irregularly shaped cavities is best performed with inelastic balloons, as elastomeric balloons tend to possess a spherical contour upon inflation. Preferential transverse dissection and asymmetrical dissection may be achieved by applying the concept of balloon eversion to inelastic balloon dissection. An inelastic balloon may contain a segment which is inverted into the central cavity of the balloon (Fig. 12.7). This segment everts outward upon

Figure 12.7
Inverted balloon concept. Both sides of the balloon are inverted into the central cavity of the balloon. Upon balloon inflation, the sides evert outward to achieve the desired final cavity configuration.

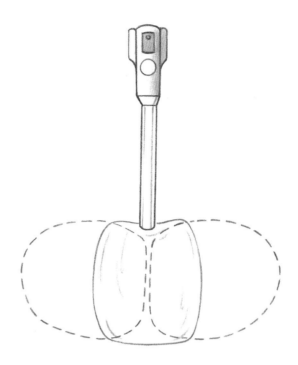

balloon inflation, progressively dissecting a cavity which matches the final configuration of the inverted balloon portion. A dissection balloon may contain one or more of these inverted segments and can extend out in multiple directions upon inflation.

Balloons may also assist in the maintenance of the dissected cavity. An inflatable dis (Fig. 12.8) may be used to lift the ceiling of the cavity, instead of the fan retractor normally employed with the mechnical lift system. The circular disc provides an increased area of circumferential lift, compared with the fan retractor, which incorporates a radial arc of 60° in the anterior direction only. In order to create an inflatable disc with sufficient rigidity to displace the flank or abdominal wall, a specialized material is used which allows the balloon inflation pressure to reach 10 psi (70 kPa). The resultant retraction surface is supportive, yet cushioned, for atraumatic displacement of body tissue. A similar inflatable disc attached to a rigid shaft may be used as a surgical retractor to support the medial wall of the retroperitoneal cavity.

A single balloon cannula may be devised to accomplish both functions of cavity formation and cavity support. One such cannula involves an inelastic inflatable wall combined with an elastomeric dissection balloon (Fig. 12.9). Following balloon dissection, the structural wall in inflated to support the dissected cavity and to seal the dissection tract for gas insufflation, if necessary. A combination of dissection and support balloons into a single cannula would make it unnecessary to exchange cannulae, removing the potential for entry into an incorrect tissue plane subsequent to cavity formation.

A second concept which combines the functions of cavity dissection and cavity support involves a multichambered balloon inserted into the extraperitoneal space, inflated to perform the dissection, and retained in position to maintain the dissected space (Fig. 12.10). A system of inflation struts on the periphery of the balloon form a dome which supports the cavity, while permitting the passage of

(a)

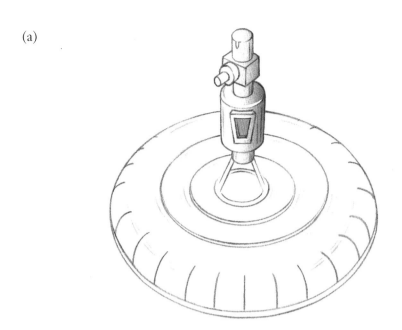

Figure 12.8
*(a) Inflatable lift balloon.
(b) The inflatable disc is
attached to the mechanical
arm to provide support for
the ceiling of the working
cavity.*

(b)

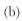

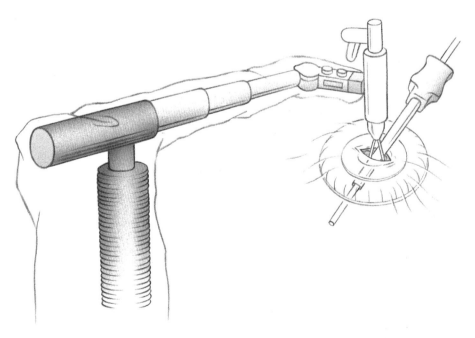

Figure 12.9
The combination dissection balloon and sealing balloon cannula. Following cavity formation, the dissection balloon is deflated and the sealing balloon is inflated to accommodate gas insufflation for cavity maintenance.

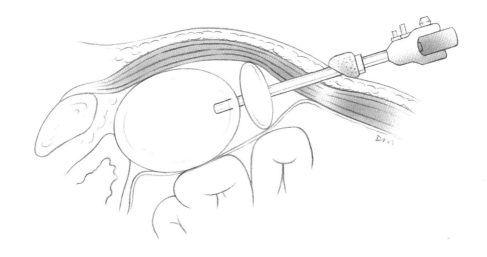

Figure 12.10
The multichambered structural balloon. The balloon combines cavity formation and cavity support functions into a single device.

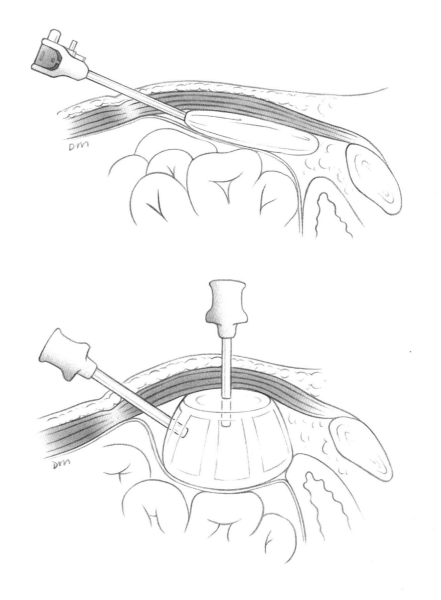

surgical instruments between the inflated structure. The structural balloon may be procedure specific, with struts arranged in predetermined sites to allow access to desired organs and anatomical regions.

Conclusion

In summary, extraperitoneal endoscopic surgery holds promise for a variety of procedures rendered difficult by bowel retraction requirements in transabdominal laparoscopic approaches. Balloon devices enable the surgeon to access and maintain specific retroperitoneal sites in a simple manner. When balloon dissection techniques are combined with mechanical retraction, additional surgical flexibility is gained. Facilitation of technical application through the development of improved instrumentation will allow the extension of minimally invasive endoscopic approaches to a wider range of procedures.

References

1 Kitano s, Tomikawa M, Iso Y *et al*. A safe and simple method to maintain a clear field of vision during laparoscopic cholecystectomy. *Surg Endosc* 1992; **6**: 197–8.

2 Newman L, Luke JP, Ruben DM *et al*. Laparoscopic herniorrhaphy without pneumoperitoneum. *Surg Laparosc Endosc* 1993; **3**(3): 213–15.

3 Chin AK, McColl MB, Moll FH *et al*. Laparoscopy without insufflation: early clinical experience. *Endosurgery* 1994; **2**: 79–83.

4 Wittmoser R. Retroperitoneoscopy: a preliminary report. In: Berci G, ed. *Endoscopy*. New York: Appleton Century Crofts, 1976: 760–1.

5 Ferzli G, Trapasso J, Raboy A *et al*. Extraperitoneal endoscopic pelvic lymph node dissection. *J Laparoendosc Surg* 1992; **2**(1): 39–43.

6 McKernan JB, Laws HL. Laparoscopic repair of inguinal hernias using a totally extraperitoneal prosthetic approach. *Surg Endosc* 1993; **7**: 26–8.

7 Gaur DD. Laparoscopic operative retroperitoneoscopy: use of a new device. *J Urol* 1992; **148**: 1137–8.

8 Keizur JJ, Tashima M, Das S. Retroperitoneal laparoscopic renal biopsy. *Surg Laparosc Endosc* 1993; **3**(1): 60–2.

9 Kieturakis MJ. Advances in extraperitoneal dissection and hernia repair. In: Arregui ME, Nagan RF, eds. *Inguinal Hernia Advances or Controversies*. Oxford: Radcliffe Medical Press, 1994: 465–73.

10 Chin AK, Moll FH, McColl MB. Balloon-assisted extraperitoneal laparoscopic hernia repair. In: Darzi A, Monson JRT, eds. *Laparoscopic Inguinal Hernia Repair*. Oxford: Isis Medical Media, 1994: 79–90.

11 Hirsch IH, Moreno JG, Lotfi MA *et al*. Controlled balloon dilatation of the extraperitoneal space for laparoscopic urologic surgery. *J Laparoendosc Surg* 1994; **4**(4): 247–51.

12 Hirsch IH, Moreno J, Gomella LG. Facilitated implantation of the inguinal reservoir of the multicomponent inflatable penile prosthesis. *J Urol* 1994; **152**: 142–3.

13 Keeley FX, Gill IS, Gomella LG. Laproscopic preperitoneal lymphadenectomy. In: Sosa E, Jenkins AD, Perlmutter AP, Albala DM, eds. *Textbook of Endourology*. Philadelphia: WB Saunders (in press).

14 Rassweiler JJ, Henkel TO, Potempa DM *et al*. The technique of transperitoneal laparoscopic nephrectomy, adrenalectomy and nephroureterectomy. *Eur Urol* 1993; **23**: 425–30.

Chapter 13

Extraperitoneal laparoscopic bladder neck suspension

G.G. Tailly, R.W. Graham, A.K. Chin and J.M. Himpens

Introduction

Female stress urinary incontinence is a sphincter-related phenomena associated with a weakened pelvic floor and hypermobility of the urethra and bladder neck, most often due to ageing and childbirth. The average urethral pressure in a standing woman varies between 40 and 80 cmH_2O, while the resting intra-abdominal pressure ranges between 5 and 10 cmH_2O. Abdominal stress situations induced by sneezing, coughing, laughing, straining, weightlifting or exercising may induce an increase of 20–40 cmH_2O in abdominal and bladder pressure [1].

During these 'stress' situations, three mechanisms are activated in an attempt to prevent leakage of urine from the bladder.

1 A reflex contraction of the pelvic floor musculature compresses the urethra and pulls it upward and forward, resulting in an increase in urethral pressure.
2 In the normal female, the retropubic position of the urethra provides for the transmission of any increase in abdominal pressure to the urethra and bladder neck, maintaining the pressure gradient between the urethra and the abdominal cavity.
3 The base of the bladder is normally its most dependent structure. If the urethra and bladder neck are well supported, maximal downward forces during stress manoeuvres will be exerted on the bladder base, rather than on the bladder neck and urethra.

In a patient with weakened pelvic floor musculature and a hyper-mobile urethra and bladder neck, the urethra and bladder neck descend, placing them in a position of greatest dependency. Any increase in intra-abdominal pressure is transmitted to the hypermobile urethra and bladder neck, causing further descent. Simultaneously, the weakened pelvic floor muscles are neither able to counteract the intra-abdominal pressure rise nor to compress the urethra and lift it upward and forward. This will result in an alteration of the normal urethral–abdominal pressure gradient, with a momentary loss of urine.

To remedy this socially incapacitating condition, a number of surgical procedures have been devised. The first procedure devised for the treatment of stress urinary incontinence was anterior colporrhaphy, described by Kelly and Dumm in 1914 [2]. Kelly's attempt to correct stress incontinence by narrowing the bladder neck via an interior vaginal approach injured a long-term success rate of only 60%. Simple plication of the vesical neck yields only a temporary repair, due to stretching of bladder neck smooth muscle over time. Modifications of the original anterior colporrhaphy prcedure exist which result in enhanced clinical results. However, the results remain highly dependent on technical considerations and tissue quality of the individual patient.

The first retropubic abdominal suspension procedure for incontinence correction was described by Marshall, Marchetti and Kranz (MMK) in 1949 [3]. In their original cystourethropexy, a suprapubic incision was used to gain access into the retropubic space. Three chromic sutures were placed through the lateral urethral wall and the adjacent vaginal wall, and anchored in the periosteum of the symphysis pubis. The crux of the operation was a return of the bladder into the pelvis and stimulation of fibrotic scar tissue that would continue to support the bladder neck. Supporting scar tissue was created by dissection of fatty tissue from the urethra, with care taken to prevent devascularization of the urethra. This procedure was the gold standard of bladder neck repair for years. Due to the placement of sutures in the paraurethral tissue, this technique involves a high risk of urethral obstruction and damage to the urethral sphincter mechanism, resulting in either prolonged urinary retention or urethral insufficiency. This problem was to some extent later avoided by placement of the sutures at a greater distance from the urethral wall. A second complication reported with this procedure was the development of osteitis pubis in approximately 0.9–10% of patients. Osteitis pubis may be a debilitating complication in an otherwise healthy woman. Severe pain in the symphysis pubis may linger on for months, with its occurence. Long-term success rates for the MMK procedure varies between 57 and 98%.

Burch [4] modified the MMK procedure in 1961 in order to provide better vaginal support to the urethra, and in an attempt to avoid the complications associated with the MMK procedure. In the Burch technique, non-absorbable sutures are placed deep in the anterior vaginal wall and anchored in Cooper's ligament. This resulted in a decreased risk of urethral injury and damage to the urethral sphincter mechanism, a decreased risk of prolonged urinary retention and avoidance of osteitis pubis. The success rate of the Burch colposuspension is 63–100%.

The pubovaginal sling operation involves the passage of a length of autologous material, such as tensor fascia lata, or prosthetic material, such as polytetrafluoroethylene (Teflon), posterior to the bladder neck. The material is sutured to the anterior rectus sheath or Cooper's ligament to form a supporting sling which compresses the urethra. The surgical approach may involve an abdominal incision, a vaginal incision, or both. Although this procedure may cure incontinence due to intrinsic urinary sphincter dysfunction, as well as stress incontinence due to bladder neck hypermobility, its potential for complication makes it an alternative choice for repair of routine stress urinary incontinence. These complications include prolonged urinary retention, erosion of the urethra or bladder, trauma to the urethral sphincter mechanism and infection of the prosthetic implant.

Needle suspension procedures combine a small abdominal incision with a vaginal incision. The paraurethral tissue is suspended from the anterior abdominal wall via percutaneous placement of sutures or wire. The procedure was first described by Pereyra [5] in 1959. A small stab incision was made in the suprapubic area and a specialized cannula was blindly passed from the incision through the retropubic space and paraurethral tissue to exit through the anterior vaginal wall. A second component of the cannula was passed from the suprapubic incision through the anterior vaginal wall at the level of the bladder neck. Steel wire was secured to the tips of the device on the vaginal side and pulled out through the suprapubic incision. The process was repeated on the other side of the urethra, and the wires tied to accomplish the suspension. In 1973, Stamey [6] introduced a suspension technique which combined cystoscopic evaluation with percutaneous needle placement to avoid needle passage through the bladder or urethra. Traction on an inserted Foley balloon catheter allowed the palpating finger to discern the proper course of the needle adjacent to the vesical neck. Suspension was performed with nylon suture. Raz [7], in 1981, described a vaginal needle suspension technique that employs more extensive dissection in the retropubic space to isolate the urethropelvic ligament and pubocervical fascia, which are looped with suture several times prior to suspension from the suprapubic region. Success rates for the various needle suspension techniques approach 90%. The advantage of these percutaneous techniques over the MMK procedure lies in their reduced morbidity and shortened operative time.

Laparoscopic techniques for treatment of urinary incontinence

Various laparoscopic techniques have been described for minimally invasive treatment of stress incontinence. These techniques utilize either a standard, transperitoneal laparoscopic approach with the establishment of a pneumoperitoneum or a total extraperitoneal form of access to conduct the repair.

A transabdominal laparoscopic adaptation of the MMK cystourethropexy was performed by Vancaillie and Schuessler in 1991 [8]. Their technique involved the placement of suture suspensions between the bladder neck and the symphysis pubis. Liu [9] described a laparoscopic version of the Burch retropubic colposuspension in 1992. His approach made use of an infraumbilical 10 mm endoscope port and four symmetrically placed 5 mm lower abdominal ports to incise the anterior peritoneum for entrance into the space of Retzius. Non-absorbable sutures were placed through the entire thickness of the anterior vaginal wall and then through Cooper's ligament on the ipsilateral side. Extracorporeal knot tying and advancement of the knot into the abdomen using a knot pusher completed the suspension. Harewood [10] used a transperitoneal approach to dissect down to the bladder neck, under laparoscopic control. A suprapubic incision is made, just short of the rectus fascia, and a Stamey needle passed through this incision to perform a double bite through the paraurethral tissue and full-thickness vaginal wall. The suture is tied over a silicone button, which remains anterior to the rectus fascia. Use of the straight Stamey needle simplifies the technique of laparoscopic suture placement. Ou *et al.* [11] developed a modified Burch technique using two strips of synthetic hernia mesh to suspend the vesical neck from Cooper's ligament. The mesh is attached to the paraurethral tissue and to Cooper's ligament with titanium laparoscopic hernia staples.

Total extraperitoneal laparoscopic approaches to incontinence surgery produce a funcitonal result similar to the transabdominal techniques described above. However, endoscopic evaluation of the procedure occurs in an operating cavity formed in the preperitoneal space, avoiding a pneumoperitoneum. Chapple and Osborne [12] reported their initial experience with laparoscopic colposuspension in 1993. A straight needle was used to accomplish the paraurethral/vaginal suspension, with laparoscopic confirmation of correct suture placement. Dissection of the retropubic space wass performed using gas insufflation via a suprapubic Veress needle. Knapp *et al.* [13] describe a technique that combines extraperitoneal laparoscopic mobilization of the bladder neck with needle suspension urethropexy. Knapp prepares the extraperitoneal cavity with balloon dissection, as originally fashioned by Gaur [14].

The authors report in this chapter a technique of total extraperitoneal laparoscopic Burch colposuspension, with balloon-assisted dissection of the preperitoneal cavity under direct visualization. Initial results have been obtained in 71 patients. This technique appears to offer a simple, reproducible method of performing minimally invasive bladder neck suspension.

Surgical technique

Position of the patient and surgeon

The patient is placed in a Lloyd-Davies position; this is a modified lithotomy position with the legs abducted but the thighs minimally flexed. This position allows good access to both the lower abdomen and the vagina. Surgical preparation is performed from the costal margin to the knees, including the perineum and the vagina, and the patient is draped. A 16F or 18F Foley catheter is introduced into the bladder and connected to a sterile drainage bag. The laparoscopic cart with the video monitor is placed at the patient's feet. The surgeon is positioned on the left side of the patient if right handed, and on the right side of the patient if left handed. The surgical assistant stands on the opposite side.

Extraperitoneal access to the retropubic space

A 2 cm semicircular incision is made on the right or left side of the umbilicus. The incision is carried down to the anterior rectus sheath, which is lifted by two Kelly clamps and incised, exposing the fibres of the rectus muscle. With an Army–Navy retractor lifting the anterior rectus sheath, the rectus muscle fibres are separated and retracted laterally to expose the posterior rectus sheath. An index finger is inserted into this incision and directed inferiorly towards the symphysis pubis. During this manoeuvre and subsequent balloon cannula advancement, care is taken not to puncture through the posterior rectus sheath as leakage of insufflation gas into the peritoneal cavity will occur. Blunt finger dissection will facilitate the introduction of the dissection balloon cannula (PDB balloon, Origin Medsystems, Menlo Park, California, USA) (Fig. 13.1). During this manoeuvre, the dissecting finger will feel the arcade of Douglas before entering into the retropubic space (the space of Retzius).

The PDB balloon is inflated slightly to test the integrity of the balloon and is prepared by lubricating the deflated balloon with a sterile gel (e.g. Instillagel or Endosgel, Farcopharma, Cologne, Germany). The balloon cannula is advanced in the tract bounded ventrally by the lifted anterior rectus sheath, laterally by the retracted rectus muscle fibres and dorsally by the posterior rectus sheath. All

Figure 13.1
The balloon dissection cannula and the squeeze bulb used to inflate the balloon.

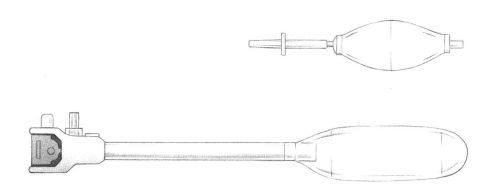

metal retractors should be removed prior to cannula introduction in case of injury to the balloon. The balloon is gently passed along the posterior rectus sheath into the retropubic space, until it reaches the pubis (Fig. 13.2). Upon contact with the pubic bone, the balloon is tilted dorsally, taking care not to push the cannula caudally under the pubic bone.

The obturator is removed from the PDB balloon end and 0° laparoscope is introduced into the cannula, taking care not to enter, and possibly injure, the deflated balloon. Using the manual squeeze bulb, the balloon is gradually inflated under direct vision (Fig. 13.3). Upon progressive inflation, the laparoscope may be inserted into the distending balloon, and one can clearly inspect the developing landmarks: the pubic bone with pubic notch, the inferior epigastric vessels, Cooper's ligament and the bladder with the prevesical fascia. The fully inflated PDB balloon is left inflated for approximately 2 minutes, then deflated and removed.

During this procedure, a 10 or 12 mm blunt tip trocar (Origin Medsystems) is prepared. The blunt tip trocar features a conical blunt tip obturator, a retention

Figure 13.2
The dissection cannula is advanced along the ventral surface of the posterior rectus sheath to the pubic symphysis.

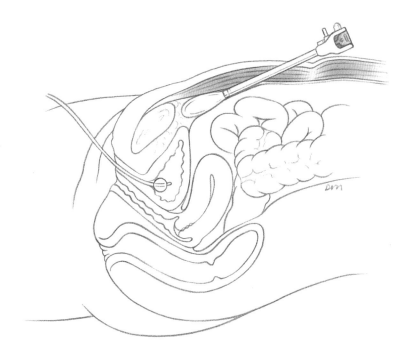

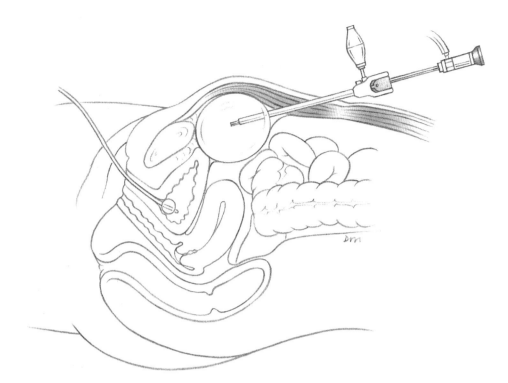

Figure 13.3
Inflation of the balloon cannula with the laparoscope inside the balloon results in dissection of the extraperitoneal cavity under direct vision.

balloon at the tip of the trocar sleeve and a foam cuff with a locking collar at the neck of the trocar sleeve. The retention balloon provides stability to the emplaced trocar, and it also serves as the internal component of an airtight seal, with the compressed foam collar serving as the external component.

After checking the integrity of the retention balloon, the blunt tip trocar is introduced in the tract vacated by the PDB balloon. The retention balloon is inflated and pulled snugly against the abdominal wall. The foam collar is advanced in contact with the skin until sufficient compression of the collar is achieved to form a gastight seal with the incision, when it is locked in place. The obturator is removed, the 0° laparoscope introduced and carbon dioxide insufflation initiated in the preperitoneal space under direct vision (Fig. 13.4).

The following landmarks are easily identified in the exposed space of Retzius (Fig. 13.5):

1 Anteriorly, the pubic bone with the pubic notch and the transversalis fascia blending into the posterior rectus sheath superiorly.
2 Laterally, the inferior epigastric vessels adherent with extensions of the prevesical fascia.
3 Dorsally, the bladder covered by prevesical fascia containing the median and medial umbilical ligaments.
4 Most often, but not always, Cooper's ligament may be appreciated.

Placement of the working trocars

Two working trocars are introduced under direct vision. They are positioned midway between the pubis and the umbilicus, just medial to the epigastirc vessels. Although two 10 mm trocars have been used, the authors most often introduce a

Figure 13.4
The blunt tip trocar is used to seal the entrance tract into the extraperitoneal cavity, which is maintained with gas insufflation.

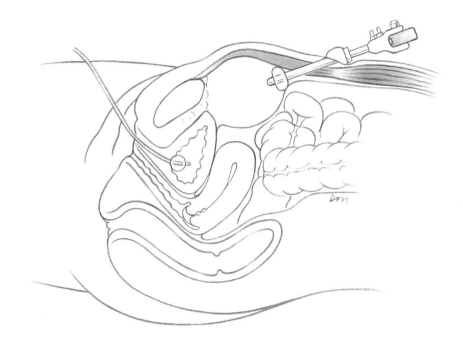

Figure 13.5
The laparoscopic view in the balloon-dissected cavity includes the following landmarks: the epigastric vessels, Cooper's ligament, pubic arch and bladder.

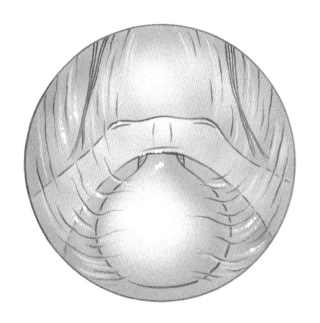

5 mm and a 10 mm port, with the 10 mm trocar placed on the side of the dominant hand of the surgeon, to accommodate the needle holder. Safety-sensing tip trocars are used (Origin Medsystems). Separately packaged sleeves available with this system allow two 10 mm sleeves to be inserted with the same obturator, providing an economical advantage. Built-in converters facilitate instrument exchanges with these trocars.

Dissection

A forceps with a peanut dissector is introduced through the 10 mm trocar, and a regular grasping forceps through the 5 mm trocar. Bimanual dissection of the prevaginal area is carried out on both sides of the urethra, taking great care not to injure the aponeurosis of the ligamentum pubourethralis which covers and supports the proximal urethra and the bladder neck. Fatty tissue along the anterior aspect of the vesical neck is clipped and cut, staying away from the periurethral tissue itself. This exposure provides adherence of the periurethral tissue to the surrounding tissue, similar to the effect achieved with the MMK repair.

Careful dissection will allow cranial and medial retraction of the bladder, uncovering the anterior vaginal wall. Elevation of the vaginal wall with a finger inserted in the vagina may enhance the dissection at this point. During this process, the inflated balloon of the Foley catheter serves as a landmark. An intermittent gentle tug on the Foley catheter may assist with orientation. Once the anterior vaginal wall has been clearly exposed on both sides of the urethra, gentle peanut dissection of Cooper's ligament is carried out on both sides. At this point in the dissection, care must be taken not to injure the branches of the inferior epigastric vessels coursing around the pubic bone at the insertion of Cooper's ligament.

Placement of the colposuspension sutures

For placement of the colposuspension sutures, a 75 cm long 2/0 Ethibond suture on a 26 mm 3/8 c needle may be used. A longer suture (120 cm length) will facilitate the performance of the extracorporeal Roeder's knot. The needle is introduced through the 10 mm trocar with the needle holder. For the inexperienced surgeon, the correct placement of the needle in the jaw of the needle holder often is the most difficult part of the procedure.

The surgeon inserts one or two fingers of the non-dominant hand in the vagina and elevates it while the assistant retracts the bladder medially and cranially. Then, with the guidance of the intravaginal fingers, the needle is inserted in the anterior vaginal wall, achieving a good bite. Next, the needle is driven through Cooper's ligament approximately 2–4 cm lateral to the midline. In order to obtain a good colposuspension, it is important not to anchor the sutures too close to the midline. Double bites in the paraurethral tissue and Cooper's ligament may be used to enhance the security of the suspension.

The needle is retrieved through the 10 mm trocar and an extracorporeal Roeder's knot is tied. A knot pusher is used to slide the knot into place. While pushing the knot into position, the inguinal vault must be kept elevated towards the Cooper ligament. Generally, it is not possible (and, provided the anchoring is performed as far lateral as possible, not necessary) to place the vaginal vault completely in contact with Cooper's ligament. Once sufficient elevation of the vaginal vault is accomplished, approximately 1–1.5 cm away from Cooper's ligament, the knot is tightened. The identical manoeuvre is repeated contralaterally. A single suture bilaterally is sufficient for a good colposuspension, but some surgeons may feel more at ease with two sutures on each side. The end result has a bat-like appearance, the wings of the bat being the suspended vaginal vaults, and the head being the balloon of the Foley catheter. Following completion of the colposuspension, a suction drain is introduced through the 10 mm trocar. The trocars are removed under direct vision and the incisions are closed. The suction drainage and Foley catheter are maintained for 24 hours. The patient is discharged from the hospital on the second postoperative day if micturition is performed without difficulty, and if the post-void residual volumes measure less than 50 ml.

One of the authors (RWG) places a percutaneous suprapubic tube and no suction drain at the end of the procedure. The tube is left open upon patient discharge form the hospital, clamped at home 48 hours postoperatively, and used to record post-void residuals. The suprapubic tube is removed during an office visit on the third postoperative day if the patient is voiding well.

Clinical experience

Between January 1993 and November 1994, laparoscopic colposuspension for urinary stress incontinence was performed in a total of 71 patients. The age of the patients ranged from 29 to 78 years, with a mean age of 52.66 years. The decision to perform a colposuspension was based on a typical history of urinary stress incontinence, physical examination, urodynamic investigation and cystoscopy.

All surgeries used the total extraperitoneal technique as an initial approach, Eleven procedures were completed transabdominally due to dense adhesions or scar formation from previous surgeries. One significant complication occurred; a patient who had her surgery converted to a transabdominal procedure developed an incarcerated internal hernia from an unclosed peritoneum 3 months after the colposuspension. She required a laparoscopic repair of the hernia. The remaining complications were minor, and included gross haematuria in one patient, urinary retention in three patients, intraoperative bleeding controlled during surgery in three patients, postoperative diarrhoea in one patient and abdominal pain/discomfort in two patients (Table 13.1).

Recurrence of urinary stress incontinence has occurred in three of the 71 patients. All three of these patients underwent repeat surgery for failed stress incontinence procedures. Two of these patient demonstrated incontinence in spite of successful bladder neck suspension. The remaining patient experienced disruption of the suture suspension. The overall success rate for this series was 96%. All patients returned to work within 2 weeks of the surgery, and nearly all patients resumed strenuous physical activities such as sports within 4 weeks.

Table 13.1
Complications from laparoscopic bladder neck suspension.

Complications	Number
Incarcerated internal hernia	1
Gross haematuria	1
Urinary retention	2
Intraoperative bleeding (controlled during surgery)	3
Diarrhoea	1
Abdominal pain/discomfort	2

Discussion

Laparoscopic colposuspension seeks to reproduce the clinical outcome achieved with conventional open incontinent surgical procedures, but with decreased postoperative morbidity. Total extraperitoneal laparoscopic colposuspension goes a step further and conducts the entire procedure outside the abdominal cavity. Advantages of the extraperitoneal approach include avoidance of postoperative intra-abdominal adhesion formation, avoidance of potential bowel injury observed with a transabdominal approach, elimination of complications associated with pneumoperitoneum and the potential for laparoscopic colposuspension under limited anaesthesia. Traditional needle suspension techniques have a decreased morbidity compared with open repairs; however, they accomplish this with the loss of direct surgical visualization. Blind needle passage increases the opporutnity for complications, including vesical and urethral injury. Endoscopy imparts visual control to the bladder suspension procedure while providing the advantages of limited incision surgery.

We have described a technique of balloon-assisted extraperitoneal laparoscopic colposuspension which seeks to simplify the procedure, reduce the operative time and provide a high degree of clinical success. Balloon dissection of the preperitoneal space is performed under direct endoscopic visualization in order to monitor correct placement of the balloon cannula and to evaluate the progress of cavity dissection. Anatomical landmarks may be appreciated during the process of extraperitoneal cavity formation, and balloon inflation yields a clean working space free of fibrous strands that remain following manual dissection of the Retzius space.

A simple balloon cannula with a foam cuff effectively seals the working cavity for instillation of the extrapneumoperitoneum. Alternatively, the preperitoneal cavity has been maintained using a fan retractor and mechanical lifting arm [15] (Fig. 13.6) to support the ventral aspect of the cavity and a laparoscopic bowel retractor to displace the dorsal surface of the cavity. Support of the working space in this fashion has permitted procedures such as total extraperitoneal inguinal herniorrhaphy to be performed under epidural anaesthesia [16]. In selected patients, this approach may be applied to extraperitoneal laparoscopic colposuspension as well. Use of a mechanical system to maintain the laparoscopic working cavity may also facilitate suture placement in the paraurethral tissue and in Cooper's ligament. Conventional open surgical needle holders may be used to place the suspending sutures as valved trocar ports are unnecessary in the absence of gas insufflation. This may further simplify the procedure, since suture placement is the most difficult technique encountered in laparoscopic colposuspension.

Decreased postoperative recovery periods and increased patient satisfaction have been noted with the preperitoneal laparoscopic approach. Early return to work and full physical activity are indications of the limited morbidity of this procedure. The high initial success rate achieved in this series is encouraging; continued follow-up will determine the long-term effectiveness of this technique.

Conclusion

The combination of a modified surgical approach and improved laparoscopic instrumentation serves to provide a successful solution to the problem of urinary

Figure 13.6
The fan retractor and mechanical lifting arm may be used to support the roof of the extraperitoneal cavity instead of gas insufflation.

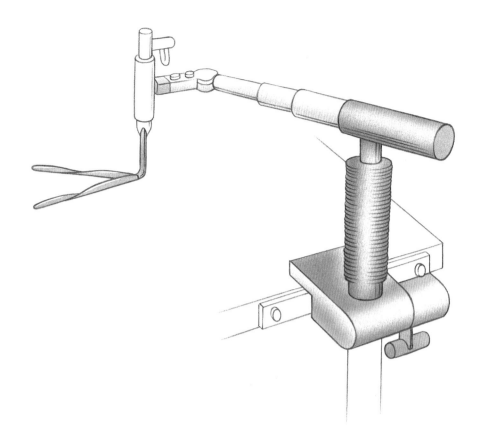

stress incontinence. Endoscopic preperitoneal dissection forms the basis for a procedure which improves the comfort level for both the patient and the surgeon. A limited recovery period and decreased postoperative pain is enjoyed by the patient, while a simplified technique and enhanced visual control is appreciated by the surgeon. Continued application and improvement of this technique will lead to optimization of a corrective approach to the misery of the urinary stress incontinence.

References

1 Mostwyn JL. Current concepts of female pelvic anatomy and physiology. *Urol Clin North Am* 1991; **18**: 175–95.
2 Kelly HA, Dumm WM. Urinary incontinence in women, without manifest injury to the bladder. *Surg Gynecol Obstet* 1914; **18**: 444–8.
3 Marshall VG, Marchetti AA, Krantz KE. The correction of stress incontinence by simple vesicourethral suspension. *Surg Gynecol Obstet* 1949; **88**: 509–13.
4 Burch C. Urethraovaginal fixation to Cooper's ligament for correction of stress incontinence, cystocele, and prolapse. *Am J Obstet Gynecol* 1961; **81**: 281–90.
5 Pereyra AJ. A simplified surgical procedure for the correction of stress incontinence in women. *West J Surg Obstet Gynecol* 1959; **67**: 223–8.
6 Stamey TA. Endoscopic suspension of the vesical neck for urinary incontinence. *Surg Gynecol Obstet* 1973; **136**: 547–54.
7 Raz S. Modified bladder neck suspension for female stress incontinence. *Urology* 1981; **17**: 82–5.
8 Vancaillie TG, Schuessler W. Laparoscopic bladder neck suspension. *J Laparoendosc Surg* 1991; **1**: 169–73.
9 Liu CY. Laparoscopic retropubic colposuspension (Burch procedure). A review of 58 cases. *J Reprod Med* 1992; **38**: 526–30.

10 Harewood LM. Laproscopic needle colposuspension for genuine stress incontinence. *J Endourol* 1993; **7**(4): 319–22.

11 Ou CS, Presthus J, Beadle E. Laparoscopic bladder neck suspension using hernia mesh and surgical staples. *J Laparoendosc Surg* 1993; **3**(6): 563–6.

12 Chapple CR, Osborne JL. Laparoscopic colposuspension — a new procedure. *Min Invas Ther* 1993; **2**: 59–62.

13 Knapp PM, Siegel YI, Lingeman JE. Laparoscopic retroperitoneal needle suspension urethropexy. *J Endourol* 1994; **8**(4): 279–84.

14 Gaur DD. Laparoscopic operative retroperitoneoscopy: use of a new device. *J Urol* 1992; **148**: 1137–9.

15 Chin AK, McColl MB, Moll FH *et al*. Laparoscopy without insufflation: early clinical experience. *Endosurgery* 1994; **2**: 79–83.

16 Ferzli GS, Sysarz FA III. Extraperitoneal endoscopic inguinal herniorrhaphy performed without carbon dioxide insufflation. *J Laparoendosc Surg* 1994; **4**(5): 301–4.

Chapter 14
Endoscopic balloon-assisted augmentation mammaplasty

M.J. Carney and A.K. Chin

Introduction

Bilateral augmentaion mammaplasty has employed a number of surgical techniques to place various types of prostheses and grafts. The augmentation mammaplasty procedure was first reported by Cronin and Gerow in 1963 [1], with the introduction of a gel-filled prosthesis via an inframammary incision. Arion [2] first described the use of an inflatable implant in 1965. Cosmetic considerations led to the development of an areolar approach to mammaplasty, reported in 1973 by Jones and Tauras [3], who employed an inferior hemiareolar incision to form a prepectoral pocket for prosthetic placement. The periareolar incision resulted in less visible postoperative scarring, compared with an inframammary incision. Concurrent to the development of an areolar approach, an axillary entry to mammaplasty was advanced by Troques [4] and Hoehler [5]. Both of these surgeons used an axillary incision to gain access for prepectoral implant placement. Removal of the incision from the mammary region results in the absence of scarring in aesthetic locations. Extension of a transaxillary approach to the placement of subpectoral prosthesis was reported by Watanabe [6] in 1982. Subpectoral implant placement is preferred by some surgeons, as it decreases the potential for capsular contracture, provides less of an obstruction to mammographic imaging and renders the prosthesis less detectable upon palpation.

Breast implants of varying compositions have been utilized over the past three decades. Prior to 1992, the standard implant incorporated a silicone rubber shell filled with silicone gel; this prosthesis was implanted in approximately 85% of all augmentation mammaplasty procedures. The gel-filled implant was preferred for its reliability versus the inflatable implant, which was assumed to have propensity for deflation. This was particularly evident in the early 1980s, when a change made in the silicone shell of the inflatable implant to improve its palpability resulted in a near total deflation rate. The situation changed abruptly in 1992 with the imposition of severe restrictions by the Food and Drug Administration in the USA on the gel implant.

Endoscopic-assisted augmentation mammaplasty

The application of endoscopic techniques to augmentation mammaplasty was conceived and developed by Johnson in 1992 [7]. Endoscopy was recognized as having the potential to decrease the morbidity of the mammaplasty procedure, while achieving a superior cosmetic result. Johnson uses an umbilical incision to initiate a subcutaneous tract on top of the linea alba and rectus abdominis fascia. A mammascope, a tubular instrument similar to a sigmoidoscope, is inserted into this tract and advanced in a straight line from the umbilicus to the medial border of the areola. A rounded obturator in the mammascope assists in its subcutaneous passage. The instrument is pushed along the abdominal surface and over the costal margin, until it enters the submammary plane above the pectoralis fascia. The obturator is removed, and a 10 mm diameter endoscope is inserted to verify the correct plane of dissection on the undersurface of the breast and to inspect the space for bleeding.

Previously, Johnson employed a 50% overexpansion of the inflatable implant to dissect the submammary pocket. The rolled up, deflated implant was inserted into the distal end of the mammascope and pushed into position underneath the breast. Subsequently, he used the inflation of a tissue expander to dissect the submammary space, reducing the possibility of implant injury due to overexpansion and excessive manipulation during the dissection process [8]. Currently, the implant is milked through the tissue tunnel after the expansion process to avoid any instrumentation contact with the implant.

More recently, other investigators have developed transaxillary endoscopic approaches to augmentation mammaplasty. Price *et al.* [9] prefer a submuscular placement of the breast prosthesis, and found endoscopy useful for controlled dissection of the pectoral muscle origins, providing predictable lowering of the inframammary crease. This group of researchers also evaluated the umbilical endoscopic approach but found themselves unable to place the implant submuscularly from this route. They noted a higher degree of control when dissection was conducted via an axillary incision. Visualization was provided by a 10 mm diameter endoscope with a 30° lens, attached to a right-angled retractor which served to stabilize the endoscope and lift the submuscular pocket. Electrocautery dissection is used to divide the pectoralis muscle and the prepectoral fascia, and to expose breast tissue in the inferior and medial borders. Lateral dissection is performed bluntly using Hegar uterine dilators to avoid cautery injury to anterolateral sensory nerves to the breast. Following achievement of haemostasis, the implant is positioned in the submuscular pocket and inflated.

Ho [10] describes an endoscopically assisted technique of augmentation mammaplasty which employs a stab incision at the lateral pole of the breast and a second incision in an apical crease of the axilla. Following blunt dissection of a retropectoral pocket, using straight and right-angled rigid probes, the pocket is distended with a glycine irrigation solution. An arthroscope with a 30° lens is used to direct an electrocautery probe which coagulates bleeding sites and divides remaining connective tissue strands suspended with the pocket. The inflatable implant is introduced via the axillary incision, following evacuation of the glycine solution.

We have introduced a technique for endoscopic augmentation mammaplasty via an axillary approach, which enlists balloon dissection in the preparation of the retroprectoral implant pocket. Balloon cannula dissection offers a simple, controlled method of separating musculofascial planes with minimal vascular disruption. It has logical application to endoscopic augmentation mammaplasty as a less traumatic and expedient means for developing the cavity for receipt of the mammary prosthesis. The device allows for improved visualization of the operative field and also acts as a stabilizer of the endoscope.

Device description

The balloon dissection cannula (Fig. 14.1) incorporates an elastomeric balloon at its distal end, and a through lumen which accommodates the passage of a 10 mm endoscope or operating endoscope. The balloon is attached in a coaxial configuration to the outside of the cannula, and it has an inflated capacity of 1 litre. The proximal end of the cannula houses a balloon inflation prot, a flap valve and a port to the through lumen that permits gas insufflation or suction aspiration if desired.

During use, an endoscope is advanced to the tip of the cannula via the through lumen, and the balloon is inflated using an inflation bulb (Fig. 14.2). Forty compressions of the inflation bulb results in the formation of a 1 litre cavity. A 10 mm operating endoscope is inserted in the lumen of the cannula to permit additional dissection in the cavity. The inflated balloon remains in the cavity during instrument dissection. The shaft of the cannula may be partially withdrawn to retract the leading edge of the balloon and create a working space, as shown in Fig. 14.3. Slight deflation of the balloon to a volume of approximately 750 cm^3 may facilitate retraction of the frontal aspect of the balloon for enhanced cavity exposure. The cannula shaft is pivoted in different directions to gain access to various portions of the cavity. Direct endoscopic visualization allows the surgeon to identify remaining bands of restrictive muscle

Figure 14.1

A schematic diagram of the balloon dissection cannula, showing the configuration of the coaxial dissection balloon and the endoscope inserted via the cannula through lumen.

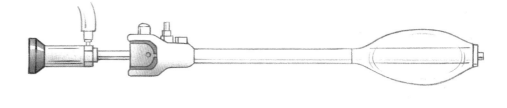

Figure 14.2

Inflation of the dissection balloon in the subpectoral space. The balloon achieves a volume of 1 litre upon inflation.

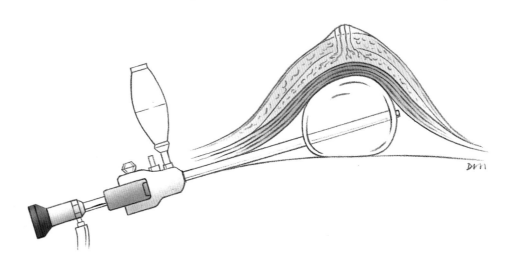

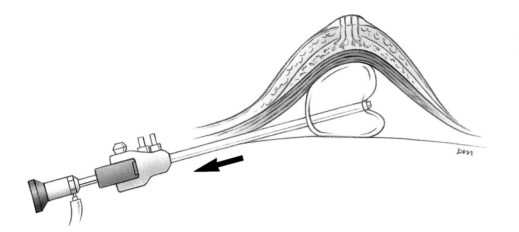

Figure 14.3
*Partial withdrawal of the
dissection cannula to retract
the leading edge of the
balloon and create an
endoscopic working cavity.*

that must be released prior to implant placement. The release occurs along the
costal margin from the level of the upper areola continuing inferiorly and
laterally to create the new inframammary fold.

Surgical technique

The procedure is carried out under general anaesthesia. A 2 cm incision is made
along a skin crease in the lower axilla and blunt dissection is performed with a
pair of curved Metzenbaum scissors to identify the lateral border of the pectoralis
major muscle. The length of the incision is mandated by the size needed to
eventually place the implant. Bacitracin solution-soaked finger-tip dissection is
used to initiate a plane in the subpectoral space. Digital probing is directed
towards the inferomedial aspect of the breast, and continued as far as finger
length permits, being careful not to disrupt the vascular perforators. The balloon
dissection cannula (Origin Medsystems, Menlo Park, California, USA) is
advanced to the distal end of the tract established by finger dissection. A 0° 10
mm laparoscope with a working channel is inserted into the device channel
through lumen of the balloon cannula. Balloon inflation is accomplished using a
squeeze bulb; the progress of the dissection is monitored using both the
laparoscope and gross inspection. Endoscopic viewing identifies the intercostal
perforators during balloon dissection, and it also provides an opportunity to
coagulate the vessels in a controlled manner. The distal pectoralis muscle fibres
are released 1 cm above the costal insertion to avoid any retraction of the major
intercostal perforators. This release occurs medially along the costal margin from
the upper level of the areola, continuing in an inferior and lateral direction
creating medial release for improved breast cleavage and inferiorly to create the
new lower inframammary fold. The rounded contour of the expanding balloon
verifies a uniform release of the pocket (Fig. 14.4).

Following dissection, the balloon cannula may be deflated slightly, and a
10 mm working endoscope advanced through the balloon cannula into the cavity.
Laparoscopic instruments are introduced through the working channel to
coagulate bleeding sites (Fig. 14.5). If additional pectoralis muscle release is
required, it is performed using a laparoscopic electrocautery tip or a laser fibre.

Figure 14.4
*A view of the dissection
balloon in position during
inflation. Uniform inferior
release is achieved by the
expanding balloon.*

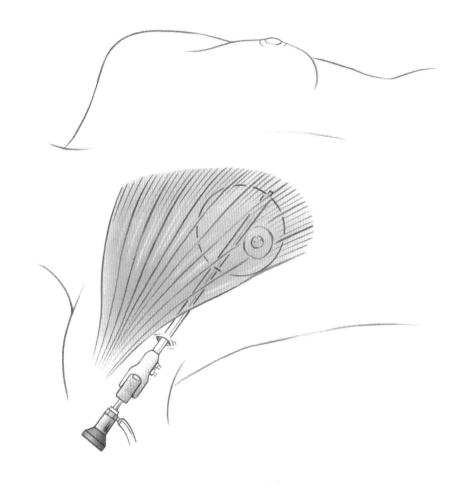

Figure 14.5.
*Insertion of an electrocautery
probe into the subpectoral
cavity. The probe is advanced
through the working channel
of an operating endoscope,
which lies in the through
lumen of the partially
retracted balloon cannula.*

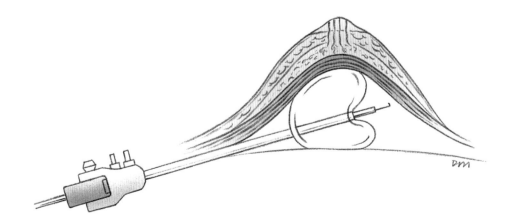

When adequate muscle release and haemostasis have been achieved, the subpectoral cavity is irrigated with normal saline. The extent of the superior, medial, inferior and lateral release are confirmed with the use of a blunt dissector. The deflated, rolled-up prosthesis is inserted into the cavity via the axillary incision and filled with a closed system of normal saline. Careful digital manipulation is used to perform small adjustments in implant positioning. The fill valve (anterior diaphragm or posterior leaf) is removed under digital control and limited visualization. Following satisfactory placement of the prosthesis, the incision is closed in two layers, using a deep closure of absorbable suture and a skin closure of non-absorbable suture. Drains may be used according to the surgeon's preference and are removed in 24–48 hours. Sutures are removed in 48–72 hours.

Clinical experience

Bilateral endoscopic augmentation mammaplasty using a balloon-assisted axillary approach was performed in 34 patients between November 1993 and August 1995. All cases except one were successfully completed endoscopically. One patient developed bleeding from an intercostal perforator which required a periareolar incision for visualization and control. The lateral location of the bleeding vessel and the rigidity of the endoscope made visualization in the intercostal space difficult via an axillary insertion site. Control of bleeding in this procedure would have been possible with the use of a flexible endoscope; however, this instrument was not available for this case. A 4 mm endoscope through a periareolar stab incision could also be used for visualization and control of bleeding.

One patient underwent unilateral repositioning of her implant to lower the inframammary fold for improved symmetry. The remaining patients had superior cosmetic results. Operative time, although initially slightly longer than comparable procedures utilizing a periareolar approach, decreased to under 1 hour towards the latter part of the series. The improvement in operative time is largely due to the decrease in time to enter into, and exit from, the subpectoral plane.

There has been no incidence of infection or capsular contracture in the limited follow-up period for patients in this series. No patients developed haematomata in the postoperative period, and all patients report normal breast sensation. The endoscopic approach has received favourable approval from all mammaplasty patients. Postoperative pain is unchanged since most of the discomfort is due to the implant stretching the pectoralis muscle. All patients were able to initiate shoulder motion the day following surgery. Patients are encouraged to start massaging the implant within 48 hours of surgery to maintain pocket size. This motion is usually limited to displacing the implant in a medial and superior direction. There are no restrictions on patient activity other than those associated with the use of narcotic pain medications.

Discussion

Development of an endoscopic transaxillary subpectoral technique seeks to achieve an optimal approach to augmentation mammaplasty, while minimizing surgical morbidity and optimizing results. Use of the technique to place inflatable saline implants is timely in the United States, due to the restriction the Food and Drug Administration has placed on the use of silicone gel prostheses. Not only is the inflatable implant the only version available for general clinical use in the USA, but it is also the design most applicable for endoscopic insertion, as the deflated implant may be rolled into a compact configuration for introduction through a limited axillary incision.

Reservations regarding the use of inflatable mammary implants have been based on limitations in reliability due to the potential for implant deflation. Changes in inflatable implant design appear to have improved the longevity of the prostheses, and recent reviews cite a deflation rate of 6% or less [11]. A large trial of the 1 year deflation rate is currently under way with results expected in 1997. Clinical consequences of ruptured or leaking inflatable implants are slight, since the saline is readily resorbed. It is anticipated that the removal of a deflated implant, a limited capsulotomy, and the insertion of a new prosthesis may all be accomplished via an axillary incision under endoscopic guidance, when required.

The transaxillary approach enables placement of the implant in a subpectoral location. Dissection of a subpectoral pocket is extremely difficult to accomplish from an umbilical approach. The distance between the umbilicus and the lower costal insertion of the pectoralis muscle increases the difficulty of entrance into the submuscular plane and its accurate release. In contrast, the axilla offers simple access to the lateral border of the pectoralis muscle, and initial exposure of the subpectoral plane may be performed under direct vision.

Subpectoral prosthetic insertion is preferred for its positive effect on implant softness, possible decrease in deflation rate and, most importantly, its lack of interference with mammography. A decrease in the incidence of a capsular contracture has been linked to a submuscular site of implant insertion by some authors [12,13]. One researcher has proposed that interposition of the highly vascularized pectoralis muscle between the prosthesis and breast tissue, which is chronicallly contaminated by bacteria, may shield the submuscular capsule from infection-induced contracture. Another hypothesis suggests that the position of the implant between two relatively unyielding surfaces — the ribs posteriorly and the pectoralis muscle anteriorly — acts to stent the capsule against contracture. In a subglandular implant, the anterior surface of the capsule is formed by soft mammary tissue which provides less resistance against capsular distortion. The ease of subpectoral access from an axillary incision facilitates this prefered approach.

Tissue dissection in the subpectoral plane may be performed by manual dissection. A blunt probe may be applied to separate the pectoralis muscle from the underlying ribs, and form the submuscular pocket. However, repeated application of mechanical probes increases the potential for increased tissue trauma and bleeding in the dissection plane. The ability to visualize the dissection process is also desirable.

Balloon dissection provides a technique for gentle displacement of tissue planes, under direct endoscopic evaluation. Balloon inflation achieves cushioned separation of the pectoralis muscle, a result of the compressibility of the air used for inflation. A subpectoral pocket is formed with minimal bleeding and endoscopic visualization confers the ability to judge the size of the dissected space.

Partial deflation of the dissection balloon left *in situ* allows additional dissection of the pocket, using an operating endoscope. Further direct visual dissection is needed to expand the surgical pocket by releasing pectoralis fibres medially and by lowering the inframammary fold. In this series, a limitation of the single axillary incision technique was observed with the inability to gain adequate visualization for haemostatic control during lateral dissection in one patient. In similar situations when the surgeon is restricted to the use of a rigid endoscope, a second incision in the areolar region may be needed to assist in the control of any retracted bleeding vessels.

The application of a single incision, transaxillary endoscopic approach to augmentation mammaplasty is also limited by the fact that approximately 40% of mammaplasty patients need to undergo some form of concurrent breast lift. Periareolar incisions are required for breast lift procedures and an endoscopic axillary approach is unwarranted in these patients.

Breast augmentation patients who do not require concomitant breast lift are candidates for an endoscopic balloon-assisted axillary approach. This procedure has had universal appeal to all applicable patients presented with the option of undergoing this procedure versus conventional open implant placement.

Conclusion

The transaxillary endoscopic approach to augmentation mammaplasty appears to provide an improved technique for the subpectoral placement of an inflatable implant. Balloon dissection of the submuscular pocket lends further assistance to the procedure by performing gentle tissue displacement under direct endoscopic visualization. The balloon also acts as a tissue retractor and endoscope stabilizer. The degree of patient acceptance and satisfaction exhibited during this early series lends encouragement to the continuation of this approach.

References

1   Cronin TD, Gerow FJ. Augmentation mammaplasty; a new natural feel prosthesis. *Trans Third Int Cong Plast Surg Washington DC* 1963: 41–9.
2   Arion H Presentation d'une prosthese retromammaire. *J Soc Fr Gynecol* 1965; **35**: 427–32.
3   Jones FR, Tauras AP. A periareolar incision for augmentation mammaplasty. *Plast Reconstr Surg* 1973; **51**: 641–4.
4   Troques R. Implantation des prostheses mammaires par incision axillaire. *Nouv Presse Med* 1972; **1**: 2409.
5   Hoehler H. Breast augmentation: the axillary approach. *Br J Plast Surg* 1973; **26**: 373–6.
6   Watanabe K, Tsurukiyi K, Fugii Y. Sub-pectoral transaxillary method of breast augmentation in Orientals. *Aesthetic Plast Surg* 1982; **6**: 231–6.
7   Johnson GW, Christ JE. The endoscopic breast augmentation: the transumbilical insertion of saline-filled breast implants. *Plast Reconstr Surg* 1992; **92**(5): 801–8.
8   Johnson GW. Endoscopic augmentation mammoplasty (letter). *Plast Reconstr Surg* 1994; **93**(7): 1527–8.
9   Price CI, Eaves FF III, Nahai F *et al*. Endoscopic transaxillary subpectoral breast augmentation. *Plast Reconstr Surg* 1994; **94**(5): 612–19.
10 Ho LCY. Endoscopic assisted transaxillary augmentation mammaplasty. *Br J Plast Surg* 1993; **46**: 332–6.

11 Rheingold LM, Yoo RP, Courtiss EH. Experience with 326 inflatable breast implants. *Plast Reconstr Surg* 1994; **93**(1): 118–22.
12 Vasquez B, Given KS, Houston GC. Breast augmentation: a review of subglandular and submuscular implantation. *Aesth Plast Surg* 1987; **11**: 101–5.
13 Puckett CL, Croll GH, Reichel CA *et al*. A critical look at capsule contracture in subglandular versus subpectoral mammary augmentation. *Aesth Plast Surg* 1987; **11**: 23–8.

Chapter 15

Equipment

N. Silbertrust

As with all endoscopic procedures, the image of the surgical site is the most important concern of the surgical team. For decades, the view through the endoscope was seen only by the endoscopist. However, in the past 10 years the use of medical video cameras has increased enormously because they provide enlarged images on multiple monitors which all members of the operating room team can view.

An integrated system is necessary to provide a high resolution, true colour image. The key element of the system is the rigid or flexible endoscope which is positioned within the body cavity. The endoscope transmits light so that the site can be viewed by the endoscope's imaging system. The image is relayed through an optical system (rigid or flexible) to the ocular or eyepiece, where it is magnified for viewing. The endoscopist can view the image directly, or, by attaching a medical video camera, view an enlarged image on a video monitor.

The author's choice for the telescopes which transmit the illumination to the site and form the image which is relayed to the eyepiece are the Karl Storz (Tuttlingen, Germany) wide angle, 10 mm diameter, 33 cm long, autoclavable rigid scopes (Fig. 15.1). Three angles of view are available: 26033 APA is 0°, the BPA is 30° and the FPA is 45°. The high resolution and large depth of field of these Hopkins rod lens telescopes are unsurpassed. The 0° and 30° telescopes are indispensable, and the 45° is often helpful.

These telescopes are introduced through trocar and cannula sets. In the past several years, endoscopic surgeons were given a choice between reusable and disposable trocars and cannulae. Lately, economic studies have shown the reusables to be very cost effective; they also eliminate the cost of inventory and

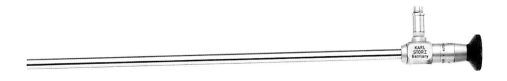
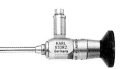

Figure 15.1
Autoclavable rigid scopes (Karl Storz).

the storage of devices before use, and the disposal of contaminated solid waste after the procedure. Examples of reusables are the Karl Storz 11 mm, multifunction trocars and cannulae (Fig. 15.2). The trocars stay sharp, the cannulae are easily disassembled for cleaning and sterilization and the multifunctional valve provides the endoscopist with a thumb-actuated valve door. There are several models of these 11 mm multifunctional trocar and cannula sets to choose from, each available in 10.5 and 8.5 cm lengths, and all with insufflation stopcocks. The trocars have conical, pyramidal or blunt tips. If, after the cannula is in place, the endoscopist wants to use a 4 mm telescope or operating instrument, a reducer (from 11 to 5 mm) can be attached to the proximal end of the cannula.

If video endoscopy is to be used, the video camera is attached to the eyepiece before the insertion of the telescope into the cannula. The light source is turned on and its level of light set, and the camera controller and monitor(s) also turned on. Usually several monitors are used so the entire staff (and students) can comfortably see the endoscopic view from the surgical site. The telescope, light

Figure 15.2
Trocars and cannulae (multifunctional valve) (Karl Storz).

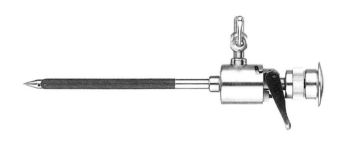

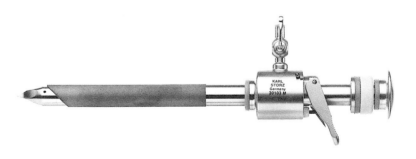

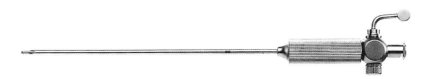

and video system are checked before insertion by viewing the back of the gloved hand from a distance of 1–2 cm.

As with all Karl Storz systems, several models of video cameras are available, each of which provides a bright, high resolution image. Cameras are all available in PAL and NTSC, 50–60 Hz and 100–240 VAC modes.

The Karl Storz Tricam is a three-chip camera which provides the maximum image quality and colour fidelity achievable in the mid 1990s. The three CCD optoelectronic chips produce over 700 lines of horizontal resolution, and are best used with high resolution monitors. The camera has an integrated zoom lens with a focal length of 20–50 mm, with function keys on the head for the control of camera functions or the video recorder/printer. Digital enhancement of the image is provided and it has S-VHS and RGB compatibility. Many other features make this the state-of-the-art video camera.

The (Karl Storz) Telecam (Fig. 15.3) is a single-chip camera which is part of a very versatile video camera system providing a choice of heads: Telecam for

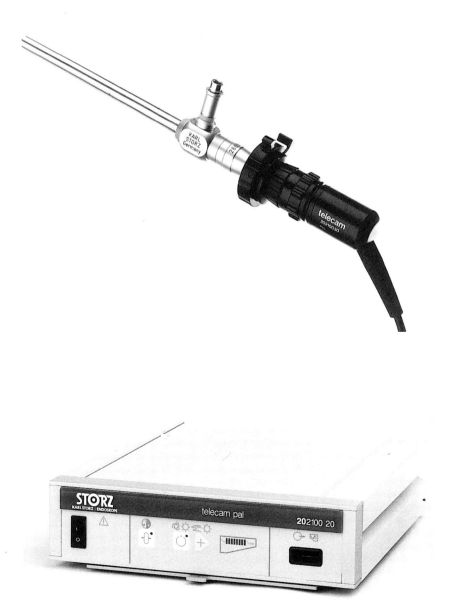

Figure 15.3
The Telecam camera (Karl Storz).

universal endoscopic use (which is ideal for retroperitoneal endoscopy) as well as camera heads specifically designed for use in urology (Urocam) or hysteroscopy (Hysterocam), with a C-mount attachment (Telecam-C) and for use on an operation microscope (Telecam-M). These heads all operate from the same camera controller which offers automatic or manual exposure control, automatic white balance, RGB and Y/C signals and a built-in character generator which is operated by a separate keyboard. The cameras have automatic zoom (25–40 mm) which is ideal for most procedures.

Video accessories are also available for the Karl Storz video systems. The Digivideo unit is a digital image processing system which can enhance the contrast of the image in real time, permitting optimal viewing of small details in the video image. Twinvideo produces two images on the same monitor by combining the images from two endoscopic cameras. The surgeon can simultaneously view images from two different directions, or from an endoscope inside an organ and another outside the organ. Or, the endoscopic image can be viewed in combination with an X-ray or ultrasound image. Images of a previously recorded procedure can also be compared to the live image, and the two images on the monitor can now be recorded together.

Many models of monitors, video recorders, character generators, colour printers and camera-to-eyepiece adaptors are also available for the endoscopic video system.

To provide maximum illumination of the surgical site, Karl Storz light sources carefully filter out a large part of the infrared and ultraviolet output of the lamps — leaving the visible light. For endoscopic surgery, we use xenon light sources (Fig. 15.4). Here again there is the choice between 175 and 300 W models. For laparoscopic surgery, we prefer the 300 W model, but we start the procedure on a low output setting and gradually increase the output to that needed for the particular procedure. Even visible light (with no infrared and ultraviolet content) can heat and dry tissue, so we never use a higher setting than is needed. The 300 W xenon light source is available with an added module for flash photography, controlled by through the lens (TTL) sensors or by manual control.

Figure 15.4
Xenon 300 W light source (Karl Storz).

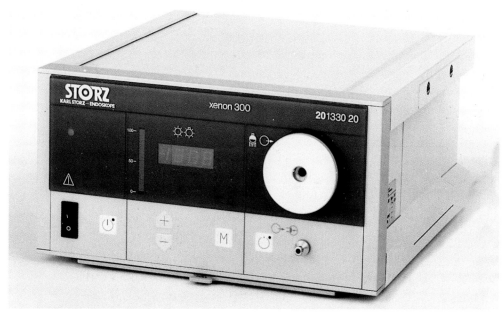

To complete the illumination system, a high quality fibreoptic light cable is needed. We use the new, longer light cables (230 and 300 cm) as their length makes positioning of the equipment easier, and the high transmission of the glass fibres eliminates much of the transmission loss associated with the older lower quality light cables.

We place the equipment associated with endoscopic surgery on a four-wheel cart, several models of which are available. The monitor is placed on the highest shelf or extension arm and other equipment (such as the camera controller, Digivideo Twindvideo, light source, pumps and insufflator) on lower shelves. With a power strip mounted on the cart and , if needed, an isolation transformer, the entire cart can be powered by one electrical cord; this eliminates the maze of cords otherwise found on the operating room floor.

To establish and maintain a pneumoperitoneum, Karl Storz has a series of mechanical and electronic insufflators for carbon dioxide (CO_2) and nitrogen oxide (N_2O) gases. We use the electronic CO_2 Endoflators, which are available in 10, 20 and 30 litre/minute models (Fig. 15.5). They work on universal power supplies and operate automatically to preset values of flow and pressure. They have input connections for a variety of CO_2 gas supplies. The 20 and 30 litre/minute units have capacities high enough to be used when the surgery requires numerous cannulae and frequent instrument changes, and with smoke evacuation. The 30 litre/minute Thermoflator (Fig. 15.6) pre-heats the gas to near body temperature, which is an advantage at high rates of flow.

Suction–irrigation pumps have proven their value over the past years for hydrodissection and lavage. The (Karl Storz) Hamou Endomat (Fig. 15.7) is a precisely controlled input–output pump which controls irrigation pressure, flow rate and suction pressure, and is electronically powered by a universal supply. Karl Storz also has CO_2-powered suction–irrigation pumps (Hydromat) with handpieces equipped with two valves for the two-pump functions (Fig. 15.8). The

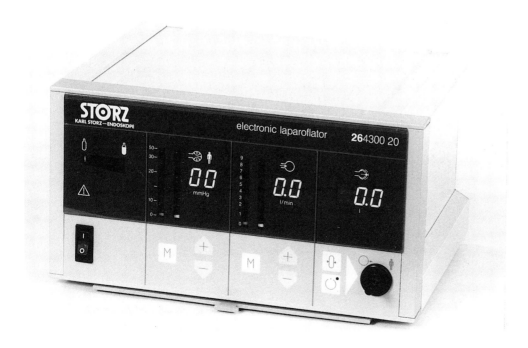

Figure 15.5
The electronic endoflator (Karl Storz).

Figure 15.6
*The Thermoflator
(Karl Storz).*

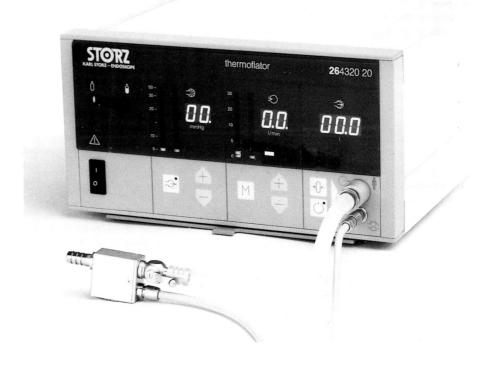

Figure 15.7
*The Hamou Endomat
(Karl Storz).*

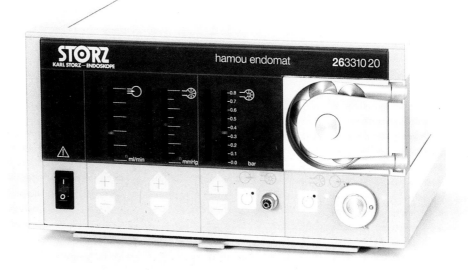

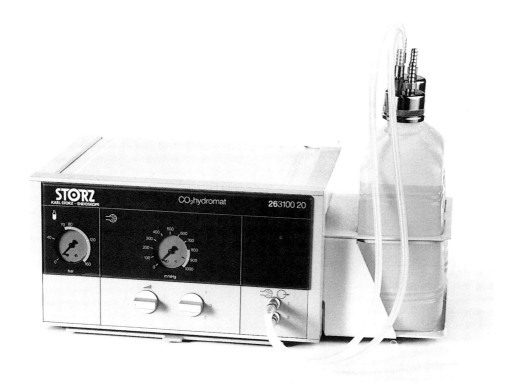

Figure 15.8
*The CO_2 Hydromat
(Karl Storz).*

irrigant can be fed from bottles or plastic bags. There is also a simple-to-use Unimat, which is an electronically powered suction–irrigation pump.

Other equipment is also available from Karl Storz for use in endoscopic surgery such as a bipolar coagulator and a high frequency generator for unipolar and bipolar cutting and coagulation. The Autocon 350 is a specially controlled high frequency generator which uses feedback circuits which measure the changing tissue parameters. This always produces the same tissue effects by varying the electrical outputs to match tissue changes.

The one remaining group of devices which is needed by the surgeon are the hand instruments. The system of endoscopic hand instruments which we use are the Karl Storz Take-aparts (Fig. 15.9). These are a series of handles and sheaths, 5 and 10 mm in diameter, into which can be inserted a wide variety of scissors, punches and biopsy, dissecting and grasping forceps. The surgeon can find in this system of rotating hand instruments all the operating tools that are needed. For instance, scissors are available with straight, hooked, Metzenbaum, curved and serrated jaws, and with insulated and uninsulated shafts. The same is true of the other instruments. Take-aparts solve the problem of cleaning and sterilizing traditional hand instruments. The Take-aparts are easily disassembled into three separate parts: the handle, sheath and insert shaft with jaws. Another clear advantage over other types of hand instruments is that a variety of inserts can be quickly and easily used with the same handle and sheath. A new sharp scissors or biopsy forceps insert can be kept on hand and used whenever necessary.

Endoscopic suturing and ligature instruments have been developed to complete the endoscopic surgeon's armamentarium. Karl Storz has led the development of these necessary instruments. The Cuschieri spring-loaded

Figure 15.9
*(a)–(c) Take-apart
instruments (Karl Storz).*

(a)

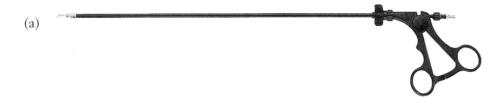

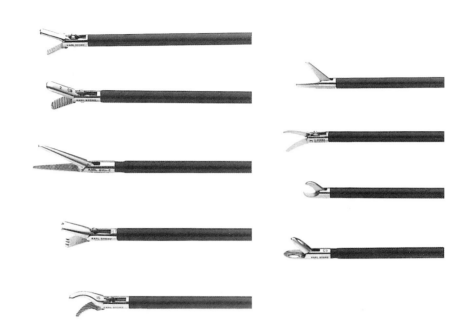

(b)

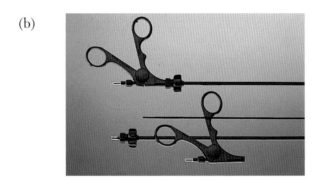

(c)

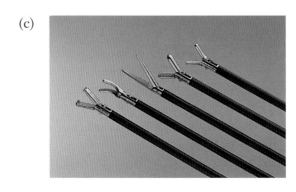

Y-handles (Fig. 15.10a) are used with a series of needle holders and suture graspers, straight and curved. The Szabo–Berci Parrot jaws and Flamingo jaws (needle holders) (Fig. 15.10b) are available for use with both 6 and 11 mm trocars and cannulae. These devices are designed with coaxial handles which makes rotation easy and which enables needle driving, suturing and the grasping of fine tissues. There are several other sets of needle holders and suture graspers, clip applications, endosuture and endoligature devices available from Karl Storz but we prefer the Szabo–Berci instruments.

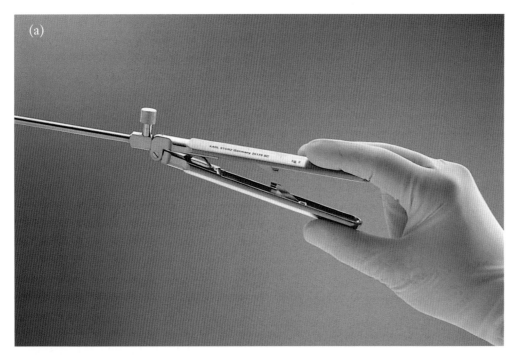

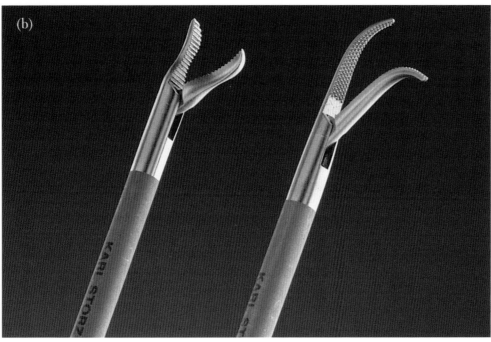

Figure 15.10
(a) Cuschieri spring-loaded Y-handle. (b) Szabo-Berci Parrot and Flamingo jaws (Karl Stortz).

Index